First Published 2023

Second Edition 2024

Copyright © Dr David Henry Dighton

Published in the UK by MediCause. 115 High Rd., Loughton, Essex. UK. IG10 4JA. All rights reserved.

British Library Cataloguing in Publication Data

A CIP catalogue record for this title is available from the British Library.

ISBN: 978-1-7385207-0-1

Book Cover by [Stefan P. From Fiverr Pro]

contents

INTRODUCTION

Have you lost a close friend or family member with a stroke, a heart attack or heart failure? That's a pity, because we can prevent or mitigate many heart problems.

Survival often hinges on knowledge which goes beyond a mere checklist of facts. These lists may overlook one crucial element – experience. Fifty years of personal experience dealing with heart problems, has enabled me to write this book and help as many would-be survivors of heart trouble as I can.

We all recognise those who are street-smart; they combine knowledge with practical experience. This makes them astute. We could say the same about those who become heart-smart. Their ability to navigate pitfalls and leverage advantages, advances their chances of survival.

Those who have seen friends and family die suddenly with heart trouble, may become concerned about themselves, but what can they do to help themselves? They will find some answers within.

Heart attacks and strokes may seem to come from nowhere, but every sudden event has its precursors, whether we are oblivious to them or choose to ignore them. This book attempts to describe when and where to look for silent heart trouble, and how to identify problems before they cause a problem.

Heart and artery diseases can present us with grave risks, many of which will remain hidden until the last minute. Would it not be better to discover the dangers before they affect us and become smart enough to mitigate them? Becoming heart-smart could save your life, but how are you to gain it?

There are many patients with heart disease under the care of doctors. If they became more knowledgeable, with a better understanding of heart trouble, could it help them put medical advice into personal perspective? I think so. Heart patients can always benefit from knowing more. They will find much about what they need to know, summarised within.

Worrying about our heart is understandable and sometimes warranted, but many harbour unfounded fears and worries. Some try to avoid anxiety; others prefer denial. Some simply hope for the best. While many are brave, others will recklessly dismiss their heart altogether!

Why should we be concerned about heart disease? That's because heart disease and cancer cause most of the middle-aged deaths in the western world. So why do so few of us take proactive steps when there are so many scientifically evaluated steps worth taking? In this book, I describe many ways to diagnose and avoid heart disease.

An awareness of danger can improve survival. Information can save lives! So let's embark on a journey to discover and learn about the heart and how it malfunctions. Your aim should be to become smart enough to answer some vital questions.

Within you will learn enough to answer questions about:

- Heart attacks,

- Dying suddenly,

- Blackouts,

- Palpitations,

- Angina, and

- Heart failure.

Heart disease may be a formidable adversary, but doesn't have to remain a silent killer.

Foremost, it is important to get familiar with the most prevalent conditions that affect the heart and circulation. There are two:

- The 'furring' process that narrows arteries (atherosclerosis) and impedes the flow of life-giving blood to heart and brain tissues.

- The effects of high blood pressure on the heart and arteries.

Within you will find brief, easy-to-understand explanations of these crucial medical conditions, together with the symptoms they lead to.

Whether you know just a little about heart problems or have some medical knowledge, this book will help you understand heart issues better.

Heart disease prevention is of utmost importance. I discuss the subject within, especially for those with heart problems in their family.

WHaT IS HeaRT DISease?

How is the heart capable beating 2.5 billion times over 70 years?

Let's start with some basic information about how the heart works. The heart is an electrically driven pump made of muscle. Oxygen from the lungs fuels its action. Small cells acting as pacemakers in the top right chamber (the right atrium) connect to other parts of the heart through the heart tissue equivalent of wires. By spreading electrical waves around the inner lining of the heart, they stimulate it into action.

Heart muscle needs oxygen as a fuel. The heart muscle gets oxygenated blood delivered by blood flowing down its own coronary arteries. They deliver enough oxygen to power the pumping and electrical activities of the heart.

Internal thickening within the inner lining of the coronary and other arteries, can cause narrowing which may eventually limit blood flow. This thickening is a type of 'furring', caused by cholesterol and calcium compound production. It is like the calcium buildup in house water pipes in hard water areas, but there is one big difference. In arteries the process is active; the 'furring' is mostly made by the inner lining of arteries (the intima). Very little deposits like snow falling on the ground. This process (atherosclerosis) is the commonest cause of heart trouble. It forms first as patches within the inner lining of arteries, referred to as plaques of atheroma.

High blood pressure (hypertension) causes another common form of heart trouble. This also narrows arteries, but in a different way. Arteries are muscle tubes with a thin inner lining (the intima) and a thin external coating. High blood pressure can reduce the blood flow in small arteries by thickening the artery wall muscle. Weight trainers know that lifting weights will cause their muscles to grow. The greater the pressure in the arteries, the more artery muscle will grow (a process called arteriosclerosis).

High blood pressure can cause bleeding from the thinner arteries that exist in the brain (a cause of strokes). There is no room for artery growth in the skull, so the arteries there are less muscular and more delicate than elsewhere in the body.

Many people believe that these two forms of artery narrowing ('furring' and artery muscle growth) are diet-related. This is only partly true. You will learn later that individual genetics play a bigger part. It is why we see both conditions running in families.

The main artery that comes from the heart (the aorta) divides into smaller branches in the same way a tree trunk progressively divides and divides again into many branches. The branches of trees end in small twigs. The arterial equivalent of these small twigs are the smallest of arteries called **arterioles**. They are just a few millimetres in internal diameter and are found in every tissue delivering the essential fuel (oxygen) for our survival. Without an adequate supply of blood and oxygen, our tissues malfunction.

Unfortunately, it is in arterioles that muscular growth narrowing occurs most, whereas the production of fatty and calcium-laden plaques occurs in arteries both large and small.

If an arteriole blocks completely, the tissue it supplies may die unless blood comes from elsewhere (other arterioles providing a collateral circulation). We use the term **'infarction'** for tissue death. When it occurs in the heart, we refer to it as a **heart attack** or **cardiac infarction.**

To summarise:

Arteries cause us trouble in two ways (causing pathological changes):

- The accumulation of fat, cholesterol, scarring, and calcium compounds within the inner lining of arteries. This is equivalent to the furring of household pipes that deliver water to our taps. In the human body, we call this 'furring' *atheroma* or *atherosclerosis*. It is patchy and inconsistent, occurring in some places but not in others. We call these patches 'atheroma plaques'.

- The second is thickening of artery wall muscle (in the small arteries called arterioles). Prolonged high blood pressure can cause the muscle walls of arterioles to grow. This can reduce flow, and increase the resistance to blood flow. It is this increased resistance to flow that raises blood pressure. In the brain, both forms of artery narrowing can cause strokes and dementia, although strokes are more commonly caused by an artery bleeding into the brain.

Despite what you may have been told, our genetics rather than our lifestyle, are responsible for most of these arterial problems. Food and exercise have an influence, but not as much as many think. (For more information on diet and the heart, read my books *HeartSense* and *Eat to Your Heart's Content.*)

The Importance of Arteries

Arteries are the pipes (muscle tubes) that carry blood and oxygen as fuel from the heart and lungs to every organ in our body. The veins return blood back to the heart. Once the tissues have extracted the oxygen to power their function, the veins carry oxygen depleted blood back to the right side of the heart. This blood looks darker than that in arteries. From the right side of the heart we pump the blood back into the lungs, where it picks up more oxygen. The blood then looks light red in colour. When we cut ourselves, the blood we see is light in colour (like arterial blood) because it contains a lot of oxygen.

The heart has two of its own arteries: the right and left **coronary arteries**. When they get 'furred' and partially blocked, angina can occur (one must be over 85% blocked). When they get completely blocked, a heart attack can happen, although that depends a lot on whether blood can reach the heart tissue from an alternative artery. When brain arteries block, strokes happen. What causes most strokes (two-thirds), is high blood pressure causing an artery to burst.

We can now detect both the 'furring' of arteries and the changes in arteries caused by high blood pressure, decades before any heart trouble occurs. Patients-to-be will often find themselves in a honeymoon period; they have no symptoms, regardless of their adverse artery changes. We have methods to detect these changes decades before any symptoms occur. By detecting these changes early, we get the chance to prevent or slow these adverse processes.

This may surprise you. Measuring blood cholesterol in individuals is not the best way to detect artery 'furring', even though the plaques of atheroma in arteries are partly made of cholesterol. There is a paradox here. In population studies, we can link the average blood cholesterol statistically to the number of heart attacks that will occur. We know it has some predictive value in populations. In individuals, however, those with high blood cholesterol may have normal arteries, and those with a low level may have obviously 'furred' arteries. Because many lives could depend on it, we need a much better test than individual blood cholesterol levels to detect the potentially lethal coronary heart disease caused by the 'furring' process. What is true for populations will not always be true for individuals, and *vice versa*.

Every year, heart and artery problems kill most middle-aged people in the western world. Prevention is possible, but for individuals detection has to come first.

Detect and Protect

Preventing some heart attacks and strokes is possible, but not everyone is interested. This is understandable given that many of us will go through life without heart or artery trouble. Many patients came to me because they had friends and relatives who had had a heart attack or stroke. They asked:

- *'Am I at risk of heart disease (could I have inherited it)?'* and,

- *'Do I have a heart problem now without knowing it?'*

Those with known heart disease should ask themselves, *'How bad is my problem?'* and, *'What needs to be done to reduce my risk of further trouble?'*

Heart Disease Symptoms

These are the important heart symptoms:

- Chest pain

- Palpitation

- Shortness of breath

- Ankle swelling

- Tiredness and fatigue.

- Blackouts

Important to Remember

- Every symptom can have several causes.

- Many patients have more than one symptom.

- Heart disease can occur without symptoms.

Symptoms usually occur when heart disease is relatively advanced. Up to that point, in the early phase of most medical conditions, there are no symptoms. This could lull many into a false sense of security.

Fortunately, for those who might have heart disease, there are clues to look out for. Many will have a history of heart disease in the family (especially angina, heart attacks and high blood pressure). Getting tested before any symptoms develop is something we should consider. This is especially important for those with a family history of heart problems.

I will detail the techniques we employ to detect early heart disease in the next chapter.

We all need to be aware of heart symptoms. Unfortunately, many people ignore them or are afraid to acknowledge them. In what follows you will find important details about each symptom.

Heart Symptoms

Chest Pain

The producers of TV and film dramas, like to portray sudden chest pain and any collapse that follows, vividly enough to shock their viewers. In reality, what happens can be quite different.

Heart attacks can be missed. They may only cause patients to feel unwell, with little else to alert them to the risk involved. There may be no pain at all.

- When patients actually get heart pain, they rarely describe it as 'pain'. They more often describe it as tightness. Sharp pains are more likely to arise from the chest wall (bone, muscle, ligament, or cartilage). The tight feeling of angina or a heart attack can simulate a band placed around the chest being progressively tightened. The main discomfort is across the front of the chest, sometimes felt in the upper arms.

- Breathlessness rather than chest pain is often the first symptom of heart disease

Many who experience genuine heart 'pain' mistake it for indigestion. Many who have indigestion think it's heart trouble. It can be difficult to tell the difference. This is because the heart and gullet (oesophagus) are in the same compartment of the chest (the middle compartment, or mediastinum). They can feel almost the same.

Palpitation

This symptom commonly induces worry, and worry can make it worse or make it last longer. Worry can also induce palpitations. Most of us will become aware of our heart beating at times. We may feel our heart:

- Beating fast.

- Beating irregularly.

- Missing beats,

- or having occasional, extra-heavy beats.

Many notice palpitation when they are at rest, especially after getting into bed.

Palpitations are often an innocent nuisance, although they may feel serious. Many get worried by them; they may even induce a feeling of impending doom. Many who get palpitations have been through a stressful period. Others are physically unfit and anxious. Fortunately, palpitation is only occasionally an indicator heart disease.

Innocent extra beats (extrasystoles) cause most palpitations. They only occasionally indicate serious heart disease.

One important form of palpitation we should never miss, is experienced more often by those over 50-years of age. It is atrial fibrillation. Atrial fibrillation causes an irregular heartbeat that is typically faster than normal. It can be so fast (over 150 beats per minute) the heart struggles to pump efficiently. The onset of atrial fibrillation can cause breathlessness. This occurs because the heart may fail to pump efficiently, allowing blood to dam back into the lungs. The lungs can become stiffer, fluid may build up, and less oxygen is absorbed. Patients will then notice some difficulty with breathing.

Read more about palpitations in Chapter 6.

Here is a link to my YouTube interview video about atrial fibrillation: www.youtube.com/watch?v=fgFJqun238o.

Breathlessness

Breathlessness ALWAYS has important implications. When it becomes noticed by the patient, we call it **dyspnoea.** Every cause needs medical attention, even if it is only induced by worry. Regard it as an early sign of heart or lung disease, and you won't go wrong.

It is most commonly caused by being overweight, being unfit, or both. Every seven pounds (3.2 kgs.) of body weight gained will cause a noticeable increase in breathlessness.

Breathlessness can be the earliest symptom of heart disease. It is more common than chest pain as an early sign of heart trouble. Be concerned if dressing makes you breathless. When an unfit older person gets slightly breathless after walking up two flights of stairs, the cause is usually unfitness and/or excess body weight. Only if it gets worse from one week to another, should one be concerned enough to get it checked.

If you have noticed your breath getting progressively shorter over short distances, get tested.

If you are breathless when lying flat, get urgent attention. This is a sign of serious heart and/or lung disease (left heart failure).

As the heart loses contractile strength (with age, coronary disease, and valve problems), it pumps less blood around the body. Blood dams back into the lungs, and fluid can collect in the feet (heart weakness is not the commonest cause of swollen feet). With more blood in the lungs, fluid may collect (causing pulmonary oedema), displacing the air and reducing oxygen exchange. Even lying still and flat in bed, patients can be breathlessness. This is the breathlessness of left heart failure (weakness of the main pumping chamber – the left ventricle).

The breathlessness of **heart failure** is often associated with other symptoms. These are: feeling tired; cold extremities (nose, hands, and feet), and swollen feet (see later).

Those who have had a cold nose with cold hands and feet for most of their lives need not worry. This condition (**Raynaud's condition**) is inherited and often noticed from the teenage years. It may not improve with age. Artery spasm, rather than heart disease, is the cause. Both medical and surgical treatments are available, but their success rate can leave a lot to be desired.

Here is a link to my YouTube interview video about heart failure:

www.youtube.com/watch?v=j31Da0Qk3xA

Other Causes of Breathlessness

- **Bronchitis:** defined as the constant production of sputum,

- **Emphysema:** (more air than lung tissue in the lungs) It can cause breathlessness at rest in older patients. There is an inherited element to it.

- **Asthma** causes breathlessness and wheezing at all ages. Paradoxically, wheezing may not be obvious when mild or when very severe. Only when it is severe will it cause distressed breathing at rest. Before that, some will notice it with minimal exercise, like dressing. It is best to get it checked since it can be life-threatening.

- **Anaemia:** Most people think anaemia causes tiredness and fatigue. This is so when it is extreme, but more often it causes breathlessness. It has to be severe to cause symptoms. Because of improved nutrition in the western world, anaemia is not as common as it was. It can occur when there has been slow internal bleeding from a peptic ulcer. Heavy menstrual periods also causes it (iron deficiency). Some will have pernicious anaemia running in their families. Although uncommon, it can be severe. Patients cannot absorb B_{12}., a vitamin necessary for blood formation. In deprived communities, anaemia can occur from malnutrition.

- **Pulmonary embolism (a clot in the lung)** is a serious cause of breathlessness. It can occur suddenly or slowly over many days. Air travel can cause thrombosis in the legs (**deep vein thrombosis**) of those prone to it. Thereafter, clots (thrombi) can travel (embolise) to the lungs. Sudden breathlessness and even collapse can result. Multiple clots, arriving to block the smallest lung arteries can slowly cause increasing breathlessness.

Clot formation can occur in association with serious diseases like cancer. It can also occur following long surgical operations. They occur especially in those who have experienced stress, those with hormone problems (the contraceptive pill, pregnancy, and menopause), and those who have a genetic predisposition to clotting.

During the Watergate affair (1972) in the US, President Richard Nixon developed near-fatal leg vein clots and pulmonary embolism.

If clotting runs in your family, get tested for clotting factors. Ask your doctor about abnormal blood factors. The Leiden Factor, PAI, and MTHFR are among those to be measured.

- **Stress: Panic attacks and anxiety are common causes of breathlessness.** Doctors remain divided about stress and its role in clotting. Many will acknowledge that stress causes hyperventilation and feelings of breathlessness. The problem is that stress comes in various forms and affects us differently. If you feel unduly stressed, consider a simple Life Change Score questionnaire evaluation (Holmes and Rahe questionnaire or equivalent). There are many questionnaires available to evaluate anxiety and depression.

- **Heart valve problems**: Mitral valve stenosis was once a common cause of breathlessness. In this case, the valve blockage does not cause heart weakness. Other valve problems can dilate the heart and cause heart failure and breathlessness.

- **Sudden changes in heart rhythm**: These can cause breathlessness, especially when the heart rhythm changes from a normal (sinus rhythm) rate of 60–80 beats per minute, to a fast rate (irregular fast atrial fibrillation, at 120+ beats per minute). This will be noticed more by those who have a weak heart already. The sudden onset of a fast rhythm can make some patients more breathless within minutes.

The Tests Needed to Investigate Breathlessness

The essentials ones are:

- A clinical history and examination.

- An ECG at rest and exercise. If heart rhythm problems are likely, a 24-hour ECG will be necessary.

- Lung function studies (breathing tests). These are useful in asthma and emphysema.

- A chest X-ray.

- If valve problems are suspected, an echocardiogram will be necessary.

Swollen Feet

Immobile people who sit for prolonged periods can have **swollen feet**. Walking around helps to pump blood around the body. The cause is mostly gravitational, and not the result of heart failure. All those with swollen feet, however, need to be checked medically for heart failure, kidney failure and hormone problems.

With the swelling of one foot or leg, one must think of infections like cellulitis (infection spreading through the skin), arthritis (gout and other forms), leg vein inflammation, and clot formation in the deep veins.

Tiredness and Fatigue

All serious medical complaints are associated with tiredness. This is mainly because many of them induce poor-quality sleep. Long-term anxiety and stress are also major causes of poor sleep, fatigue, and exhaustion.

As we become ill, we get tired. The body burns lots of energy while fighting disease and maintaining failing bodily functions; energy reserves diminish and tiredness follows. The tiredness caused by illness is not easily reversed by natural sleep. In contrast, the tiredness associated with late nights and working long hours is readily reversed. The cure for normal degrees of tiredness may lie in changing life circumstances.

The consequences of long-term tiredness, fatigue, and exhaustion can be serious. I have often seen a connection between energy depletion, heart disease and stroke in some patients. This is how it might work for some:

When a person is energetic, increases in their motivation and stress will increase their performance. As they fatigue, their performance no longer improves and remains flat. When a fatigued person is pushed, their performance will diminish further, and they will head towards exhaustion. When we are exhausted, our personal energy has been burned out, and sudden changes in our overall medical condition can become a risk. Like elastic stretched towards its breaking point, our medical condition can suddenly change or snap. By 'snap' or 'change', I mean a sudden, dangerous change in a bodily function like blood clot formation or a change in immunity (with pneumonia and other infections like COVID seen to occur). In exhausted patients, heart attacks and strokes can result from rapid clot formation or bleeding.

This explains why regenerative sleep is so important to health.

As the heart weakens (heart failure), many patients experience increasing tiredness. Physical inactivity, increased worry, diabetes, and the effects of some drugs like beta-blockers and diuretics, can make it worse.

Blackouts (Syncope)

Fainting is the commonest form of blackout (or syncope) doctors see. Fainting is rarely serious. It can, however, be a sign of early pregnancy, an undiagnosed illness, or a stressed state.

The problem is that fainting can be difficult to differentiate from the other causes of altered consciousness: epilepsy and the onset of very slow heartbeats ('heart block' requires a pacemaker to treat it). Sudden, fast heartbeat problems (ventricular tachycardia and fibrillation), are potentially life-threatening causes of blackouts.

Blocked heart valves only rarely cause blackouts (a severely blocked aortic valve can cause them). Blocked or 'furred' arteries in the neck can, however, promote clot formation and cause strokes (with clots traveling to the brain). More often, multiple mini-strokes can cause transient symptoms like altered consciousness, facial numbness or weakness, an inability to enunciate words, or transient weakness in an arm or leg. Small clots forming in the neck arteries can break off and travel within the arteries to the brain (cerebral emboli). They can cause transient ischaemic attacks (TIA) and small strokes.

The Tests Required for Blackouts:
- An ECG at rest.

- A 24-hour heart rhythm monitor recording.

- Exercise testing, and

- If epilepsy is suspected, brain tracings (EEGs) will be required.

THE SIGNS OF HEART DISEASE

After being interviewed by your doctor with your present medical history, past history, family history, social history and treatment history being noted, the next crucial step is to examine your body. These fundamental steps are essential for an adequate clinical assessment, except in exceptional emergency circumstances. To ensure correct and acceptable management, all the information gathered from your history and examination is vital. A doctor's ability to select the relevant information from this wealth of data is an art fuelled by knowledge and experience. Even in technologically advanced specialties like cardiology, the doctor-patient relationship plays a significant role in enhancing the process. If you find yourself not being interviewed or examined, it is important to question why. If you receive answers like, "too little time" or you encounter obvious disinterest, seek a second opinion.

Your examination should start in the doctor's reception area, although you may have to wait until you enter the consulting room. How you walk and your general demeanour will be noted. Whether or not you look unwell, is of vital importance. It will prove important if you are breathless and have pale or blue lips. When shaking hands, your doctor can judge the temperature of your hand and note whether your fingers are white or blue, cold or warm. These simple observations can be made before any word is spoken. If your doctor knows you well, changes in your condition should be obvious. Continuity can be a vital feature of medical practice, but it has slowly become accepted as irrelevant and less important clinically. I cannot, however, overemphasise the advantages of continuity for the patient doctor relationship.

When examined for heart disease, expect your doctor to feel your pulse and note whether it is slow or fast, regular or irregular. Each characteristic can imply a specific diagnosis. More advanced features can prove useful. For instance, the shape of your pulse waveform could allow suspicion of an outlet valve (the aortic valve) restriction (aortic stenosis).

It is important to observe the veins in your neck. The pressure in these veins will be raised in heart failure and reduced in dehydration. The major arteries in the neck deliver blood to the brain. They (carotid arteries) are felt on both sides of the neck beneath the jaw. Their pulse waveform can help detect a severe blockage in an artery or valve; only severe blockages are detectable, however.

Moving to examine your chest while you are sitting, your doctor will want to listen to your heart and lungs. The valve sounds (and murmurs) are best heard with a stethoscope at the front and left side of your chest. Your lungs are best heard on either side, front and back. Doctors may ask you to take big breaths and to hold your breath at various stages. From these examinations, doctors can detect valve narrowing, valve leakage and lung diseases (like asthma and emphysema). Tapping the chest is one way to assess lung resonance. Resonance increases when emphysema is present (the lungs are more full of air); it decreases when fluid collects around the lungs (pleural effusion). Your heart can be more easily felt when you lay on your left side. A hand placed over the area can assess the position and size of the main pumping chamber (left ventricular), and the force of its contraction.

Your body is full of blood-supplying arteries. Feeling the pulses in your abdomen and legs is sometimes important.

While standing, your doctor may want to look for varicose veins in your legs and swollen feet. If foot swelling is present, the next question is whether it dents under finger pressure (after pressing for 10–15 seconds). We call this pitting oedema (caused by fluid in the tissues). If the skin dents under pressure, prolonged sitting (gravitational oedema) and heart failure are both possible diagnoses.

The temperature of the feet and nose can be relevant in heart trouble. As the heart gets weaker and pumps less efficiently, the skin temperature of the hands, feet, and nose can drop. Many people have permanently cold extremities (Raynaud's condition related to artery spasm), so one must not assume that their heart is weak.

Tenderness of the calf muscles is sometimes a sign of deep vein thrombosis (DVT) and a potential cause of breathlessness (from clots passing to the lungs: pulmonary embolism). The context is important. DVTs occur after operations, accidents, and with prolonged stress. They can occur in prolonged serious illnesses like cancer, but also in pregnant women, and those taking the contraceptive pill or hormone treatment for menopausal symptoms.

Heart Tests and Their Value

After taking your history, and your physical examination is complete, the next step will be to request tests (investigations). Traditionally, we use them in medical practice to confirm the diagnoses made so far. More than ever, investigations are being used to replace a full history and physical examination. In those cases that are difficult to diagnose, this is a major cause of error. Except for some emergency situations, do not agree to investigations without your history and examination being completed.

The tests used to evaluate heart disease are:

- ECGs (electrocardiograms)

- Exercise ECGs

- 24-hour ECGs

- Blood tests

- Echocardiograms (mostly from the chest wall, but sometimes from the gullet, when it is called trans-oesophageal
  echocardiography).

- CT scanning.

- MRI scanning

- Isotope scanning.

- Cardiac catheterisation used to

(a) take X-ray pictures from within the heart and arteries, and

(b) to assess the heart's electrical system (electrophysiology).

I will briefly describe each of these tests, why we do them and their
expected relevance.

An ECG

This is an electrical recording test invented in the 19th century.
It is sometimes used to reveal what is happening to the mechanical
functioning of the heart. It more easily detects electrical defects, heart
rhythm disturbances, and drug effects, although it can sometimes
suggest heart muscle functioning problems. ECGs can be difficult to
interpret, and few doctors other than cardiologists seem confident
about it. One reason is the occurrence of normal variants among the
many abnormal patterns. Many doctors rely on computer-based AI
recognition for ECG diagnosis, but this can be subject to error if the
clinical context is missing.

The Exercise ECG

ECGs taken before, during, and after some exercise are the equivalent of a car road test for the heart. Most cardiologists use a treadmill

for the exercise; some still use exercise bicycles. With a patient walking on the treadmill, both the slope and speed can be adjusted. In common use is a fixed protocol, where the speed and elevation of the walkway can both be increased every three minutes (the Bruce protocol). Exercising for a minimum of nine minutes is usual for those of average fitness. This will usually suit young and middle-aged ambulant people. We can modify the test to accommodate athletes, and those challenged by exercise.

The ECG during and after exercise is used to reveal signs of coronary artery narrowing, but the narrowing usually has to be greater than 80% before the test becomes positive. When the effects of artery narrowing are not revealed by an ECG after exercise (a false negative), other important clues lie in observing a patient who develops chest tightness, breathlessness or fatigue. Ideally, all exercise tests are attended by a doctor or someone specially trained to observe the test, and to interpret its outcome.

The 24-hour ECG

This is a very useful test for detecting what is happening during blackouts or when patients experience palpitations.

The patient wears a small recording device fixed to a waist belt. The ECG leads (wires) are attached to the skin of the chest and connected to the device. The device will then record an ECG continuously for long periods (24–72 hours with a Holter recording). Other devices available can transmit the patient's ECG to a receiving centre, where a technician can analyse it as it is happening.

There are other ambulant recording devices. When we think longer recordings are necessary (to capture rarer cardiac events), we can implant recording devices under the skin.

A reduced form of ECG can now be transmitted using a mobile phone. There are also event recorders. These work with a recording loop rather than with continuous long-term recordings. The patient stops the device just after any event that troubles them. The loop recording can then be accessed and played back to see what was happening during the event (palpitation or blackout). For convenience, the recording can be transmitted down a telephone line to a specialist centre for analysis.

Blood Tests

There are many tests that aim to predict the occurrence of 'furring' and clotting in arteries. They are much more useful for detecting population risk than individual risk. The very best of them is HDL, or 'good cholesterol'; the worst of them are total cholesterol and triglyceride levels. We know that free fat (triglyceride), LDL or bad cholesterol, homocysteine, C-reactive protein (CRP), and the clotting factor fibrinogen, all have some value when assessing population risk. Population averages allow us to define targets for lipid (fat)-lowering therapy. None of them reliably predict the presence of fat formation in a patient's arteries, occurring as it does in those with coronary artery disease. Rather than guessing, we can use direct imaging of the cholesterol 'furring' within arteries using ultrasound and CT scanning.

Blood tests are good for detecting the heart damage that occurs during, and shortly after a heart attack (during which heart tissue damage occurs). We use both blood troponin and cardiac enzyme levels for this. If you find yourself in an A&E unit with chest pain, thinking you may have had a heart attack, doctors will request a blood test looking for raised levels of troponin. The higher the levels, the more damage the heart has suffered. We must do the tests within a certain time window; not too soon or too late after any chest pain starts.

Echocardiogram

In echocardiography, we use the sonar principle of sound reflection to visualise the interior of the heart. The ultrasound it uses is both produced and detected by the same hand-held transducer. The ultrasound used is harmless to both adults and babies in utero. The echoes that bounce back from heart tissues help create computer-generated images from inside the heart.

The device allows us to image how valves move. Using this technique, we can measure heart wall thickness and the size of each heart chamber, as well as detect the extent of heart muscle damage caused by a heart attack.

We have put another principle of sound physics to good use. As a noisy car or train approaches, the pitch of the sound we hear increases. As it passes, the pitch wanes. This is the **Doppler effect**. Using the Doppler principle, we can visualize blood flow (moving towards or away from the transducer), and measure the severity of narrowed and leaking valves.

Echocardiography cannot be used to visualize the whole length of the coronary arteries; they are too small. Sometimes their place of origin from the aorta can be glimpsed, but not much else.

As an extension, and improvement of the ECG exercise test, we can combine it with echocardiography. We can do echocardiograms and ECGs before and after exercise (or a stimulant drug infusion for those unable to exercise). Changes in pumping chamber contractions are sometimes detectable (**stress echocardiogram**). Sometimes the heart muscle is normal at rest, but does not contract normally on exercise. When this is seen, it can successfully detect coronary artery disease.

All medical machines and devices developed over the last 40 years have become progressively smaller. Many now incorporate diagnostic AI programs.

CT (Computed Tomography) Scanning

As opposed to plain, one-shot X-rays, this technique acquires 2-D pictures and can compute 3-D information. Although reduced greatly over the last fifty years, radiation exposure remains a downside.

The 'furring' in arteries is mostly a mixture of three main components, one of which will usually predominate. These components are cholesterol, scar tissue, and calcium-containing compound (calcium apatite not chalk). The latter can block X-ray transmission. In this way, we can get pictures of the extent and position of the calcium present in the coronary arteries. We can then calculate a score for the total amount of calcium present. This score (the Atheston or Coronary artery Calcium [CAC] Score) is low or zero in those with minimal or no coronary artery disease, and high (over 300 or 400) in those with a coronary artery narrowing problem. The position of the calcium present can be of vital importance. Coronary disease in the front arteries (anterior descending branch) is usually more serious than 'furring' found in the other artery branches (right coronary and the circumflex or posterior descending). In this way we can assess future cardiovascular risk.

A cardiac CT scan is a valuable screening test for those suspected of having coronary disease; especially for those with suggestive symptoms, a strong family history, and/or abnormal results of an ECG exercise test. When convinced that the patient has coronary disease, we usually proceed directly to a coronary arteriogram rather than bother with CT scanning. We can then do stenting and other procedures at the same time.

For cases of intermediate certainty, a **CT angiogram** is useful. Dye injected at the same time as a cardiac CT scan can show major restrictions in coronary blood flow. The image quality is not as good as those taken during coronary angiography.

CT angiography has the advantage of not being invasive. We need not insert tubes into arteries as in coronary arteriography. A problem with both tests is the potential for radiation damage. This depends on the radiation doses used. Even with the much lower doses now used, we prefer not to repeat these tests too often.

MRI Scanning

We can repeat magnetic resonance imaging as many times as we like because no radiation is involved. We can use it when echocardiography fails to provide adequate images of the heart and major blood vessels in the chest.

For many years after its invention, the equipment was too slow to capture moving pictures of the heart. MRI machines have become faster and faster, along with many software improvements. The technique has proven excellent for defining the defects of congenital heart disease, the imaging of large blood vessels (looking for aortic aneurysms and dissection), and for assessing heart muscle for damage, muscle disease (cardiomyopathy), and rare heart tumours.

MRI scanning can present a problem for the claustrophobic; they will have to spend quite a time lying in a metal tube. Ask to be tested in an open scanner if this could be a problem for you.

Isotope Scanning

These are tests that aim to measure heart muscle functioning. The heart will not function normally if coronary artery blood flow becomes blocked (narrowed coronary arteries) or if there is extensive muscle damage (after a heart attack).

Heart tissue concentrates some radioactive isotopes (thallium, technetium, gallium, and iodine). Each will last a different length of time in the body. During that time we can see how well blood is being delivered to the heart and how much is taken up by heart muscle. We can take images at rest and after exercise. Comparing the two allows differentiation between normal tissue, irreparably damaged tissue, and heart tissue receiving a restricted blood supply.

Patients can have either coronary disease with artery narrowing or a healthy blood supply. A sufficient blood supply implies a low risk of future events. The presence of an alternative blood supply (from another artery), called a collateral circulation, is one reason for this. With additional arteries present, fewer patients would be at risk of heart attacks. Their presence can mean the difference between life and death. For this reason, a lot of research has been directed toward discovering the mechanisms responsible for extra artery growth. The hope is to find a drug that will encourage collateral artery growth. If that were possible, some bypass operations might become unnecessary.

For those who want more technical information, go to www.msd manuals.com.

Positron Emission Tomography (PET Scanning) is a recent addition to the imaging techniques available. By injecting radioactive glucose, it is possible to get an insight into the metabolism of heart muscle. Using rubidium allows the assessment of coronary flow. It may become possible to see if the artery 'furring' is actively growing or dormant. The active ones are those most likely to attract clots, block a coronary artery, and cause a heart attack. Because of their high risk, these arteries might be considered for stenting before any symptoms develop.

Cardiac Catheterisation

This is an invasive technique. It involves introducing small-calibre tubes (catheters) into the veins and arteries of the arms or legs. We can guide catheters to the heart under X-ray control (fluoroscopy), and position them in each heart chamber and in each coronary artery. We can measure pressures, assess valve function, and take X-ray videos (angiograms) of heart chambers and coronary arteries.

Visualisation of the coronary arteries has been available since 1958. Lower-dose X-ray machines, and softer catheters, have made the procedure safer.

Cardiac catheterisation is required for the acquisition of detailed information. The technique allows us to put artery stents and new valves in place at the same time.

Not all catheters are tubes; some are plastic-coated electrical conducting wires. By introducing them into the heart chambers, the electrical activity of the heart can be assessed (electrophysiology). The technique is also used to implant pacemakers and to deliver microwaves (ablation) when treating some fast heart rhythm problems.

BLOOD Pressure Problems

Two important facts to consider:

High blood pressure is the commonest cause of strokes.

Low blood pressure predisposes to fainting.

Many people inherit **low blood pressure**, but it can also result from taking drugs given for high blood pressure. It is associated with athleticism, and made worse by a low salt (sodium) diet. Low blood pressure has been made more common by the gradual reduction of salt in our diet (to avoid high blood pressure).

Those who inhabit the rain forests of the Amazon and Borneo have some of the lowest average blood pressures recorded. Low blood pressure needs to concern only those who faint frequently. Consistent low blood pressure has an advantage. It reduces the risk of hemorrhagic stroke (caused by bleeding into the brain). Low blood pressure can present a problem to doctors managing patients with heat stroke, septicaemia, and heart trouble. Under these circumstances, it relates to heart and circulation malfunctioning.

High blood pressure has two causes:

- Blood flow restriction in tiny arteries (arterioles) is the first cause. Muscle growth of the artery walls restricts the blood flow. We call this **primary hypertension**. The increased resistance to blood flow, caused by widespread artery wall muscle growth (arteriosclerosis), raises the pressure of the blood flowing through them. These arterial changes are genetically driven, so those with no family history of high blood pressure are much less likely to develop permanent high blood pressure and strokes. Transient high blood pressure can happen without artery wall thickening; blood pressure can be normal one minute and raised at another. This we call **labile blood pressure**.

- Rarer causes of high blood pressure (secondary hypertension) result from kidney disease and hormone problems (adrenaline, cortisol, and those associated with the menopause and the contraceptive pill). Some hormones raise blood pressure because they cause salt and water retention. Eating lots of sodium salt can make blood pressure higher, but only in those prone to it. Those who consistently have low blood pressure can benefit from added salt, especially with the extra salt loss that occurs with sweating in hot climates.

What is high blood pressure? The World Health Organisation (WHO) defines it as blood pressure (BP) above 140/80. Others define it as that above 130/80. What do these numbers mean, and how is blood pressure generated?

If we insert a small tube into an artery and attach it to a pressure measuring device, pressure waveforms for every pulse can be seen. The way we usually take blood pressure is much less accurate. We measure it using a machine (sphygmomanometer) with an inflatable cuff placed around an arm (or leg). Whatever the method of measurement, the peak of the pressure wave is called the systolic blood pressure (140 millimetres of mercury [Hg]). This is the top pressure generated by each heartbeat. The lower figure we call the diastolic pressure (80 millimetres of Hg). This is the pressure in every artery between heartbeats (the resting pressure). All the arteries taken together resemble a blood-filled balloon; like any inflated balloon, the elastic walls exert an inward pressure.

We measure blood pressure in everyday clinical practice by squeezing an arm (or leg), until the blood flow in the arteries stops. The pressure in the cuff will then equal the maximum blood pressure within the artery (the systolic pressure, or the top figure in the BP measurement). The lower pressure (the diastolic) is more difficult to measure. As we slowly deflate the blood pressure cuff, the sound heard over the artery (with a stethoscope) will change from sharp to dull. At that moment the pressure dial will indicate the lower (diastolic) resting arterial pressure.

The errors made while measuring blood pressure are considerable; this makes recording it as accurately as 122/65, scientific nonsense. What we should record is something like, a blood pressure lying between 120 and 130 (systolic), and 80 to 90 diastolic. Besides any machine related error are errors caused by the natural variation of blood pressure. It varies from one moment to another, from one minute to another, and from one time of day to another. These considerations make 'ball park' figures more acceptable. It would make better sense to record a BP as low, normal, variable (sometimes high, sometimes low), or consistently high, but common sense remains in short supply.

Each beat of the heart has its own top (systolic) and lower (diastolic) pressure, and that presents yet another problem. Which beat and which pressures are we to take as representative? Let's assume the heart beats 70 times every minute. That would be 70 x 60 beats per hour (= 4,200 beats per hour); that equals 24 x 4200 beats, or 100,800 separate blood pressures every day. The problem is that we usually only take blood pressures a few times each day. So which of these few measurements should we take as representative, given that the stresses and strains of life can cause considerable variation in blood pressure? Perhaps an average would be better? We can do this, but it is not routine.

As the heart beats, it generates pulsatile blood flow and a pressure wave at the same time. Measured using a column of mercury (now the outmoded method of old-fashioned blood pressure machines), the top (systolic) pressure in the example above would be equal to the pressure generated by a 14cm (140mm) column of mercury in a vertical glass tube. With the heart fully relaxed between beats, the pressure in the arteries would equal that of a column of mercury 80mm (8cm) high. Mercury is dangerous stuff, so mechanical devices (aneroid sphygmomanometers) have now replaced the old machines.

There is yet another accuracy problem. Using the same blood pressure cuff, more pressure is needed to compress the artery in a large arm, than in a thin arm. Pressures taken from large arms thus require higher pressures to compress the artery. For this reason, I would often take the blood pressure of those with large arms, using their thinner forearm. We partly solve the problem by using different cuff sizes. Using a large cuff on a small arm can result in pressures that are falsely low, and using a small cuff on a large arm can result in pressures that are falsely high (compared to the pressures measured using a needle in an artery). Make sure your doctors and nurses use the right size cuff for your arm. Question them if you think the cuff they are using is too small or too large. If you do not, you may end up with a false diagnosis of high or low blood pressure when it is normal.

It's a good idea to take your own blood pressure. Buy a machine that you can use on your upper arm. Avoid wrist machines and those with printers (many will lose the little tickets they print)! Take at least three consecutive readings each time, and keep a diary of your blood pressure results. Many get anxious, even while taking their own blood pressure, so discard all the first readings.

Twenty-four-hour BP monitors are available that attach to a waist belt. This can take the patient's blood pressure (and ECG if necessary) every half hour. Blood pressures can be recorded over 24 or 48 hour period, during both effort and relaxation. Although somewhat disturbing, blood pressure measurements can be taken during sleep. 'Real' high blood pressure will usually remain raised during sleep.

The problem with consistent high blood pressure (blood pressure for which treatment is advisable) is that it can cause our organs to change. Any adverse changes in our arteries, heart or kidneys need to be monitored. At the same time as our heart muscle and arteries thicken, the artery walls within our brain may thin, making them more fragile and liable to bleed. When this happens, a **hemorrhagic stroke** will occur. Artery clotting, with small clots flying off (emboli) to block a brain artery, will cause **embolic strokes**.

High blood pressures caused by anxiety, alarm, and stress (like 'white coat' syndrome) will not usually cause organ changes. We believe this type of high blood pressure to be transient (labile blood pressure), and the result of reflex responses, during which adrenaline-like chemicals are released at nerve endings.

When trying to decide which blood pressure is 'real' ('primary hypertension' that needs treatment) and which is 'labile' (transient high blood pressure that requires no treatment), doctors face a diagnostic problem. To resolve the problem, we can look for changes in the body caused only by 'real' hypertension. Patients with this type of blood pressure must seriously consider having their risk of stroke reduced by taking anti-hypertensive medication.

The changes in the body caused by hypertension are:

- Heart muscle growth. The main pumping chamber (left ventricle) gets more muscular (left ventricular hypertrophy). This is detectable using a chest X-ray, an ECG, heart ultrasound, and MRI scanning.

- The muscle walls of small arteries (arterioles) become thickened (arteriosclerosis). We can see this at the back of the eye (the only place where arteries are directly visible). The thickening sometimes restricts blood flow to the kidneys, resulting in a slow deterioration in their function (evaluated with blood tests, etc.). This can cause hormone changes that potentiate hypertension. Restricted blood flow in the brain is one cause of dementia (vascular dementia).

The more heart muscle thickens, the more likely the patient will be to have a hemorrhagic stroke. We need an accurate measure of heart muscle thickness to assess the risk a patient faces from high blood pressure (this does not yet feature in NICE guidelines as a necessary routine). I found it helped my patient management decisions.

For anyone with high blood pressure (hypertension), there are some important questions to answer:

1. Has my heart muscle been affected? Hypertension can make it grow; this is called hypertrophy.

2. Has it affected my arteries (thinning in my brain, thickening in my kidneys)?

3. Is my blood pressure high all the time, or just when I am worried or stressed?

These questions are important because the answers help assess the risk of hemorrhagic stroke and kidney damage (the most dangerous consequences of high blood pressure).

The Treatment of High Blood Pressure

It is important to reduce the chemical angiotensin (a precursor of adrenaline) in the kidneys and elsewhere.

So-called ACE (angiotensin converting enzyme) inhibitors, and ARBs (angiotensin re-uptake blockers) are drugs that can lower blood pressure and stop heart muscle and artery wall growth.

Their generic or chemical names (as opposed to the trade names, vary from country to country). Those ending in '-pril' are ACE inhibitors (like lisinopril, enalapril, etc.); those ending in '-sartan' are ARBs (like losartan, candesartan, etc.). They work by blocking or reducing the amount of adrenaline production in the body.

Other drugs treat high blood pressure in other ways. Some dilate the arterioles or smaller arteries (these we call alpha blockers). The blood pressure drops because dilated arteries offer less resistance to blood flow. Drugs like amlodipine do this. Because of increased flow, many develop swollen feet. Felodipine acts similarly.

We commonly prescribe diuretics for high blood pressure treatment. They make the kidneys excrete more water and sodium salt in the urine. The combination of taking a diuretic, hot weather, and a low dietary salt intake (now fashionable) has become a common cause of fainting.

As a lifelong fainter with low blood pressure myself, I have always eaten salty food (or added salt to my food), especially when exercising in hot weather. Salt has helped me elevate my low blood pressure to normal levels. Those with high blood pressure who eat extra salt risk increasing their blood pressure. Those prone to high blood pressure should avoid extra dietary salt intake.

If you are taking any drug for high blood pressure, refer to the accompanying drug leaflet for the list of side effects. Note which are rare and which are common.

Remember that 60% of all those taking any prescribed drug will have some related adverse symptom.

Stress and Alcohol

Some resistance to medication may be found in those who have been stressed for a long time. Their high blood pressure can be difficult to treat. Away from the stress, their blood pressure will sometimes return to normal, even while taking no medication. Treating their blood pressure successfully may need to include solutions to their stressful problems. If that proves difficult, rest and relaxation, more holidays, yoga and sedative drugs, all have their place.

Alcohol can lower blood pressure. Just occasionally, it explains why hypertension becomes resistant to treatment. We should always re-assess blood pressure control after a heavy drinker takes little or no alcohol for one week. Some will find it unacceptable to stop drinking, even after accepting an increase stroke risk.

Heart Murmurs and Valve Problems

Before and during the Second World War, it was thought dangerous for schoolchildren with heart murmurs to exercise. No man with a heart murmur was eligible to join the armed forces. The assumption was that a murmur meant a weak heart; a heart that shouldn't be strained by physical activity. We now know this was mostly incorrect policy.

What causes a heart murmur?

Murmurs (a whooshing heart sound heard through a stethoscope) come from narrowed (stenosed) and leaky valves. Holes in the heart (between the heart chambers), and open channels near the heart, can also produce loud murmurs. There are four heart valves, two of which (the mitral and aortic valves) are responsible for most murmurs.

Rheumatic fever once caused many of the valve defects diagnosed by doctors. The problem began with a streptococcal throat infection, followed 10 days after by arthritis, carditis (heart inflammation), nephritis (kidney inflammation), and sometimes encephalitis (brain inflammation). Rheumatic pains and the swelling of different joints were common, hence the name rheumatic fever. Some patients passed blood in their urine (nephritis). Rarely, patients developed writhing, uncontrolled arm movements (St. Vitus' Dance), caused by brain inflammation. Although inflammation of the heart valves, joints, kidneys, and brain could occur together, it was joint swelling that most troubled patients.

By a strange coincidence, the antibodies created by the body to inactivate the streptococcal throat bacteria also attacked joints, heart valves, the kidneys (nephritis) and brain tissues, inflaming each to a different extent. Once a common disease of childhood before the 1960s, rheumatic fever is now rare in developed countries. In over 50-years of practice in the UK, I saw only two cases.

The loudest murmurs are those caused by narrowed aortic valves (main outlet valve) and leaking mitral valves. The mitral valve separates the top and bottom chambers on the left side of the heart (lying between the left atrium and the main pumping chamber, the left ventricle). Other loud murmurs are made by holes connecting the right and left pumping chambers (ventricular septal defect, or VSD). Apart from these loud sounds, there are many more subtle valve sounds, some of which are very quiet. The correct evaluation of all these signs will enable a doctor to make the diagnosis, and assess the severity of valvular heart trouble. Unfortunately, not all doctors find it easy to hear the more subtle sounds. Few medical students left our undergraduate teaching course at Charing Cross Hospital, capable of identifying and interpreting the key heart sounds and murmurs. It is usually only advanced students, who make a special study of the subject, who become capable.

Heart murmurs result from mechanical defects, but not all mechanical defects produce murmurs. A hole between the top chambers of the heart (an atrial septal defect) will often go unnoticed because the blood passing through it makes no appreciable sound. If any defect causes the heart to enlarge and become weak, an operation to repair the defect may be warranted. In some cases (like aortic valve narrowing and leakage), it is often wise to operate before any symptoms develop. With other valve problems, we do operations to relieve symptoms. It is for cardiologists to decide which valves are causing the symptoms.

For many decades now, we have replaced heart valves using open-heart surgery. The latest trend is to replace them using a catheter technique (tubes inserted through the veins and arteries). Not all patients are suitable for this less-invasive technique. It is a question that those with valve defects need to discuss with their cardiologist and cardiac surgeon.

Valve problems are mostly assessed using echocardiography. Much less frequently now, do we need to investigate further using heart catheterisation. Introduced in the late 1960s, I was one of the first, with Graham Leach, to use echocardiography in the UK (at St. George's Hospital, London SW1). This painless test uses high-frequency ultrasound to image arteries, the heart, babies in the womb, and many other internal organs (like the gallbladder, etc.). It involves no more than placing a microphone-like probe on the skin of the chest. The probe produces the ultrasound and then listens for the reflected echoes.

Ultrasound is used to visualise valves, to measure heart wall thickness (in high blood pressure), and image the interior lining of arteries as they thicken with cholesterol, scarring, and calcium formation (atherosclerosis). This harmless imaging technique can be repeated as often as necessary to follow the progress of valve defects, atheroscle-rosis, and heart wall thickness (to see if our treatment has prevented heart muscle change or stopped the progress of 'furring'). Ultrasound tests are now seen as essential for the early detection and management of cardiovascular disease.

If you have a valve problem that needs an operation, many surgeons will want to image your coronary arteries; depending on your age and symptoms. They may consider a coronary angiogram or coronary CT angiogram necessary before any operation.

Heart Rhythm Problems

Those who feel palpitation (missing beats or beating fast) usually have a heart rhythm problem. Most of them are harmless and are often associated with anxiety, consuming caffeine containing food products, drinking too much alcohol, and unfitness. If faintness and blackouts accompany palpitations, they are more likely to be serious and in need of urgent investigation.

Many will experience at least one episode of palpitation during their lifetime. Extra heartbeats interrupting the normal, regular rhythm of the heart for one or two seconds, is the usual cause of the symptom. Noticing palpitation can itself cause anxiety, trepidation, and even panic. Some anxious people will hyperventilate, and this will further exacerbate the problem. A few come to fear for their life. Anxiety and fear cause the body to produce adrenaline-like compounds, and it is these that can worsen heart rhythm disturbances. Any of these influences on palpitation can make them feel worse, increase their number, or make them persist for longer. In such cases, a doctor's first job will be to calm the patient and explain the nature of the problem.

We all release stress hormones (cortisol and adrenaline) when under duress. Noradrenaline is the substance released by the nerve endings attached to the heart. They make it speed up and sometimes produce extra beats (extrasystoles). When given intravenously, similarly acting drugs cause the heart to beat faster and heavier, and sometimes to beat irregularly. Some notice palpitation only when their normal regular rhythm is replaced by an irregular one.

When I was a young junior doctor working in cardiac research, I gave patients small intravenous doses of isoprenaline (an adrenaline-like substance) to test their pacemaking function. I noticed that the heart rate changes of nervous patients were exaggerated compared to those who were calm. Anxiety and tension seem to increase the sensitivity of the heart to adrenaline and other stress hormones. For this reason, beta-blockers (drugs that block adrenaline) are very useful in the treatment of anxiety-driven palpitation. Stress management and improving athletic fitness will also help some with mental health issues.

Extra beats (extrasystoles) are mostly innocent and will only rarely arise from heart disease. This is not an assumption, however, that any patient with palpitations should make. Extra beats are more often felt when going to bed. This is because blood flows back to the heart when lying down. Patients who are underweight feel them more readily than those who are overweight. As well as caffeine drinks, alcohol and tobacco, some pharmaceutical drugs cause them. The drugs in cold remedies (some contain phenylephrine), and those given for asthma are common culprits. Cocaine use has become more common, and with it some will get extreme, uncontrolled palpitations. This will occasionally risk the lives of those using it.

Reassuring patients is not always easy since the symptom can feel genuinely serious. Since they occur more often in stressed, anxious, and unfit people, they can become yet another thing for them to worry about.

A constant fast heart rate with irregularities mixed in, sometimes causes palpitation. One in particular that concerns doctors is atrial fibrillation (the atria are the top chambers of the heart). I have found this to be more in those over 50-years of age. Age-related, microscopic scarring within the upper chambers of the heart (the atria) is the usual cause. Instead of the heart beating regularly, the top chambers of the heart (the atria) shimmer or fibrillate, rather than contract regularly. Chaotic electrical waves arising from several places in the top chambers cause it. The electric waves reverberate just like water in a bath after it has been disturbed. When this happens, blood flow into the main pumping chambers (the ventricles) becomes less than with regular atrial contractions. This can lead to breathlessness and a worsening of angina (in those who already have it).

Atrial fibrillation hides a potentially serious risk. Without a regularly beating heart, small clots can form on the inner walls of the atria (the two upper chambers). These sometimes detach and shoot off (embolise) into the lungs (pulmonary embolism) or brain (cerebral embolism). Cerebral embolism is one cause of strokes and mini-strokes (TIAs, or transient ischaemic attacks). For this reason, we advise all patients with atrial fibrillation to take an anticoagulant drug (like apixaban). These reduce the risk of clot formation and have been shown to prevent strokes.

There are other electrical heart problems that cause palpitations. A few people have extra electrical pathways connecting one part of the heart to another. They are present from birth, and come with many variations. They have exotic names like the Wolff Parkinson White syndrome and the Levine Lown Ganong syndrome. We can diagnose most of them using ECGs and by introducing electrical wire catheters into the heart (electrophysiology). We can microwave any extra pathways found and inactivate their electrical activity. The technique is called electrical ablation.

Routine Testing for Palpitation

Most times, testing with an ECG or a 24-hour ECG will define the type of palpitation or tachycardia (fast heartbeat) troubling the patient. Dysrhythmia is the term we use for all these rhythm disturbances.

An exercise test will sometimes yield extra information. When exercise suppresses extra beats, they are usually harmless; when exercise makes them worse, we must assume they are dangerous. We then strongly advise further testing.

An echocardiogram is useful for assessing palpitations. It can help diagnose those associated heart valve and heart muscle problems that sometimes cause them. The important anatomical features we need to measure are heart chamber sizes. Stretching of the heart chambers is an important associated feature of palpitations like atrial fibrillation, although the underlying cause of the rhythm is the microscopic scarring (progressive fibrosis with age) of the electrical pathways in the atria.

BLACKOUTS anD PacemaKers

There are three forms of blackout:

- Fainting. Internal reflexes cause low blood pressure and a slow heart rate (vaso-motor syncope).

- Those caused by sudden heart rate changes (from normal to slow or very fast).

- Epilepsy.

Even for experienced experts, it is sometimes difficult to decide which is which.

The commonest form of blackout is fainting. Fainting results from reflex action, through nervous system pathways that connect the heart to the brain. Nerve fibres exist that allow the automatic control of the heart rate and blood flow in both arteries and veins (these nerve fibres form the autonomic nervous system). This specialised part of the nervous system can slow and speed the heart when necessary, and control the blood flow in the smaller arteries and veins.

William Harvey, a famous English physician living in the 17th century, tried to find out why exercise and emotion speed the heart rate, and why relaxation and sleep can slow it. He never found the answer. The discovery of the autonomic nervous control system had to wait for the English physiologist, John Langley, who discovered and named it in 1898.

In those prone to it, unpleasant experiences can induce fainting. Some who experience pain or an upsetting sight, can precipitate an internal reflex that slows their heart, lowers their blood pressure, and diverts blood from their brain. Sweating and pallor (a pale skin) will usually occur at the same time. Low blood pressure reduces blood flow to the brain., and can cause various levels of altered consciousness. In most people, the onset of fainting is gradual (one might observe them becoming vacant, pale, and sweaty). Just occasionally, the process unfolds rapidly and results in profound unconsciousness.

Those who are deeply unconscious may need cardio-pulmonary resuscitation (CPR). If the patient is deeply unconscious (rare), they may need a thump on the chest to reverse the process. If that doesn't work, some further CPR expertise may be needed.

The required treatment for a slow-onset faint is less dramatic. NEVER sit them up, or bend them over with their head between their knees. Lay the person flat. If possible, arrange their feet and legs above their head level. If they are semi-conscious, ask them to move their feet up and down from the ankles in order to exercise their calf muscles. This will pump venous blood back towards their head.

Something similar can happen to diabetics, especially those who have injected themselves with too much insulin or have failed to eat soon enough afterwards. The episode is not a faint, but can look like one. The cause is a low blood sugar (hypoglycaemia). Before they become fully unconscious, and as quickly as possible, give them either glucose or some table sugar, preferably in liquid form. Tablets, chews and gels are also available for this purpose. One must NEVER pour fluid into the mouth of someone who is unconscious.

Patients who are subject to fainting only rarely need a pacemaker. Those who do, will usually need one that stimulates the top and then the bottom of their heart in a normal sequence (two chamber pacing).

When they were invented in the 1960s, pacemakers were the same size as a basic hamburger (one from that renowned worldwide fast-food chain). They are now much smaller; the size of a large coin or medal. The pacemaker unit contains a battery, with electronic circuits generating regular pulses to stimulate the heart. We implant pacemakers under the skin, but they can still communicate with outside sensing apparatus via a radio link. Functional pacing data can be stored in the device and most pacemakers can now be programmed remotely (when to pace and when to stop pacing). All the stored data about how the pacemaker has functioned can be downloaded.

We usually implant pacemaker units under the skin, somewhere near the armpit. We connect the pacemaker unit to a plastic coated wire electrode, once we have advanced it through a nearby vein into the interior of the right heart. The tip of the electrode must touch the interior of the heart (the endocardium), in a place where it is unlikely to move. We usually perform the procedure under local anaesthesia. A skilled operator can accomplish this in less than 30 minutes. When I was teaching doctors to do it, it sometimes took them hours. From a time before Hippocrates (before 370 BC), a big part of medical training has always been apprenticeship. Not all apprentices will find initial favour with their master, and not all will ever find favour with their patients.

Implanted pacemakers come in many varieties, all of which function for years before they need replacing. With regular checking, impending battery failure can be detected, and a new pacemaker inserted. This requires the spent pacemaker box to be removed and replaced with a new one under local anaesthetic.

Slow Heart Rate Blackouts.

Typically found in those older than 70 years, are sudden blackouts that can come without warning. An electrical blockage that has taken years to develop, can suddenly cause the heart to be beat, half as fast as normal. The normal transmission of electrical activity is blocked half-way between the top and bottom of the heart. The heart can stop momentarily or beat very slowly. The pumping chambers will usually start to beat at their own intrinsic rate (usually less than 40 beats per minute). We refer to such sudden attacks due to electrical heart block as **Adams-Stokes'** syncope (blackout). The insertion of a pacemaker to stimulate the heart will overcome the problem. We can program them to work when the heart rate drops, and to switch off should the rate return to normal.

Because it comes with little or no warning, Adam-Stokes' blackout can put a patient's life in jeopardy. This is especially true when they occur while driving or walking in a hazardous place. Patients are not allowed to drive until a working pacemaker is implanted. Patients with pacemakers will set off airport and other alarms, so they must carry proof of pacemaker implantation with them.

Fast Heart Rate Blackouts

These usually result from heart disease. We now know that apparently fit people and athletes can collapse because they have undiagnosed heart muscle disease (cardiomyopathy). Any patient with a serious heart problem will face a similar risk. When heart disease is the cause, a blackout will occur when the heart pumping chambers become suddenly chaotic electrically. The ventricles appear to shimmer or fibrillate (**ventricular fibrillation, or VF)**, while pumping no blood at all to the brain. The patient will be unconscious, have no pulse, and will have stopped breathing. A sudden collapse from VF could signal the end of their life, unless someone skilled in cardio pulmonary resuscitation (CPR) is at hand.

Before any catastrophe occurs, some heart patients will be lucky enough to have short bursts of transient VF recorded. Monitoring in hospital and 24-hour ECG recordings might show it. Patients may then be eligible for a life-saving defibrillator, implanted in much the same way as a pacemaker. They are designed to detect VF and thereafter to shock the heart back to normal rhythm. They do this by generating a short, but powerful pulse, of electricity. Although this can be life-saving for the patient, it can be a very unpleasant experience for them. Once patients have experienced a shock, they will usually try to avoid another (avoiding undue exercise, emotion, alcohol and drugs).

Epilepsy

There are many types of epilepsy. Fits (involuntary convulsive movements) do not characterise every type. Some cause vacant attacks (temporal lobe epilepsy), blackouts, and other states of altered consciousness. Many patients with epilepsy have experienced a premonition of an attack, but many episodes occur with no warning. They can occur at any place and time. In contrast to those who faint, epileptics are not usually pale and sweaty. In addition, their pulse can be normal or a little faster.

An electrical brain tracing or EEG recording (electroencephalo-gram) is used to help with the diagnosis. Recordings may need to be done with the patient awake and while asleep. In newly diagnosed epileptics, we often do an MRI brain scan to exclude a causative tumour. If one is found, removal can cure epilepsy.

The commonest treatment for epilepsy remains anticonvulsant medication. Under development are newer techniques, like deep brain electrical stimulation and laser-guided ablation.

Many epileptics are barred from driving, but there are exceptions to be considered.

Rare Heart Problems

Heart Muscle Disease

One heart condition that hits the news occasionally is cardiomyopathy. The sudden death of a young athlete or notable person, will make the headlines. An inherited form of heart muscle disease is often responsible.

There are several types of heart muscle disease, but the hypertrophic sort (where the heart muscle becomes bulkier) is well-known to doctors. At a microscopic level the muscle fibres of the main pumping chamber (the left ventricle), are disordered and prone to electrical instability (extra heartbeats, ventricular tachycardia or ventricular fibrillation). Heart muscle can grow abnormally and block the outflow circulation of blood from the heart. This we call **hypertrophic obstructive cardiomyopathy or HOCM** for short.

Other types of cardiomyopathy (heart muscle disease) cause the heart to weaken. The heart dilates, the muscle walls thin, and the heart volume expands, expanding like a small balloon This is **dilat-ed cardiomyopathy**. The basic problem lies within the microscopic structure of the heart muscle. Because medical treatment may not be good enough, some of these patients become eligible for heart transplantation.

We can detect cardiomyopathy early using echocardiography, al-though this is rarely used in routine health screening. I introduced it for my patients 25-years ago and found only three unsuspected cases. Patients asked me why we didn't routinely screen their heart in this way, given its vital importance to life and death. Explaining that we would only rarely discover a problem was unacceptable to most of them. They wanted their car checked to ensure that the wheels were not about to fall off, and their brakes were not about to fail them. Their concern was *whether they had a heart problem or not*. This attitude contrasts with national healthcare policy; decisions are made by committees and based on what is cost effective for the population.

We often advise family screening for cardiomyopathy because heart muscle disease can be inherited. The prognosis and management of those family members found to have it, must be discussed with each patient.

Treatments range from medications that help symptoms, and those that stop complications like fatal rhythm problems. Some patients may be suitable for surgery, including heart transplantation.

Those with enlarged hearts often need treatment for heart failure. There is a simple physical reason for this. Try to squeeze a broom handle. Now try squeezing a large tree trunk. The pressure you can generate decreases as the circumference increases. Small hearts pump better than large dilated hearts because they can generate more pres-sure.

We need detailed technical evaluations when evaluating cardiomy-opathy. They include echocardiography, 24-hr ECG recording, and MRI scanning, etc. They must be done before deciding which treatment approach is appropriate.

Aneurysms

Long ago, when car and bicycle tyres had inner tubes, it was not uncommon for a bubble or 'blowout' to appear on the wall of a tyre or inner tube. The bubble would appear at a weak spot. To avoid sudden rupture, tyre repair or replacement had to be done. Something similar occurs with arteries, especially those in the abdomen (abdominal aortic aneurysm), chest and brain. We consider removal of those in the abdomen when the blowout or arterial aneurysm grows to greater than 5cms in diameter. If it has grown over a short period (over months or 1-2 years), removal may become urgent.

Within the chest, in the upper aorta, such artery enlargements can be very dangerous. They usually form a more complicated type of aneurysm (dissecting aneurysm). Blood can track between the layers of the artery wall, splitting it (dissecting it) as it grows. As more blood collects in the newly created space (the false lumen), it presses inwards, reducing the amount of blood able to flow through the main channel (the lumen) of the artery.

High blood pressure and artery 'furring' both predispose to aneurysm formation.

The splitting effect within the artery wall can cause severe, sudden onset, chest and back pain, for those with a dissecting aneurysm. Doctors may not diagnose it until someone with experience suspects it. An osteopath once referred two patients to me. He suspected that both had more than just rheumatism and arthritis. The presence of high blood pressure and back pain together, prompted his concerns. Both patients had early dissecting aortic aneurysms.

We now have CT and MRI scans to help us diagnose aneurysms quickly. Aneurysms in the upper chest require urgent major surgery to replace the defective arteries with artificial ones. This is high-risk surgery, best done in the specialised centres where they perform it frequently. Urgent action can be life-saving.

Pulmonary Hypertension

This is high blood pressure in the lung arteries – the pulmonary arteries. The lung circulation, and that of the rest of the body (the systemic circulation) are separate. Blood flows around the pulmonary system to pick up oxygen, then goes on through the systemic arteries to circulate oxygenated blood throughout the body. One large pulmonary artery arises from the right ventricle and then divides into two. Right and left pulmonary arteries deliver blood to each lung. A separate form of high blood pressure in the lungs (pulmonary hypertension) is rare. It is associated with the restriction of blood flow to the lungs. Four percent of cases have no discernible cause. We refer to this as **primary pulmonary hypertension**. Because it has serious consequences, it usually requires highly specialised care. Conditions like emphysema, pulmonary embolism, and heart valve narrowing (mitral valve stenosis), left sided heart failure, and holes in the heart can all cause high blood pressure in the lungs (secondary pulmonary hypertension).

Bacterial Endocarditis

A blood infection that goes on to destroy heart valves is the cause. A serious infective illness will usually accompany it. The correct name for it is septicaemia; now commonly referred to as 'sepsis'. The diagnosis often presents difficulties for doctors. Long-term infective illnesses with no obvious cause always present a diagnostic problem. The first step is to think of endocarditis as a possible diagnosis. It will then be necessary to grow the bacteria in the blood, and to look for valve thickening or valve damage on an echocardiogram.

We once assumed that dental extraction was the cause. Bacteria from the roots of teeth were thought to enter the circulation when we extracted them, and would thereafter settle on heart valves where they would cause swelling and damage. For this reason, patients with heart valve problems (those most at risk) used to receive large doses of penicillin before any dental intervention. The commonest bacterium involved (streptococcus) has remained sensitive to penicillin-based antibiotics.

The guidelines we are now supposed to follow, dismiss any close relationship between dental infection and endocarditis. As a result, preventative penicillin is no longer advised routinely, although there are exceptions. I would continue to follow the old policy for anyone who had endocarditis previously.

Some guidelines, all of which are based on large populations, will not apply to some individuals. I liked to discuss the guidelines and the risks with each patient, and to adjust their management accordingly. Because a doctor's job could be in jeopardy (regulators are constantly looking for dissenters), few will want to risk my policy in these matters, even if they agree with it.

Genetic Diseases

Some aneurysms result from those genetic diseases which affect the elasticity of arteries. Marfan Syndrome is one such condition. I have only seen 3 cases. Patients are unusually tall, thin, and double-jointed. Their joints and sinews are looser than normal (double-jointed) and they have eye problems. A similar condition is Ehlors Danlos syndrome. I have also seen only two such cases.

Other rarely encountered genetic diseases are:

Inherited Tachycardia (Fast Heart Rates): Brugada syndrome, and Long QT syndrome. We diagnose them initially using an ECG.

Arrhythmic Right Ventricle: I found this in a few athletes after their unexpected collapse. Underlying it was right heart muscle disease, predisposing the individual to ventricular tachycardia and fibrillation.

See the chapter on *Inheritance and the Heart* for more examples.

Inflammatory diseases

Serious inflammatory diseases can sometimes affect the heart. Rheumatoid arthritis, and lupus erythematosus, are examples. They can adversely affect the arteries and valves of the heart. Fortunately, osteoarthritis, the commonest cause of joint trouble, does not.

There are many quite rare congenital heart conditions that affect children and adults. We usually diagnose them later in life (adult congenital heart disease). I will describe some of these next.

congenital Heart Disease

Many pregnant mothers are concerned that their baby might be born with an abnormality. When they occur, there are many reasons. Genetic defects, inadequate diet, rubella in pregnancy before 12-weeks' gestation, the mothers' age, diabetes, alcohol, tobacco (and secondary smoking), and some drugs have all been implicated.

Most congenital abnormalities are difficult to understand without some knowledge of foetal anatomy and development, so only a simple description is possible here.

The more severe foetal abnormalities will not always be compatible with life. Foetuses that have multiple abnormalities may spontaneously miscarry in the early days and weeks of gestation. When babies survive pregnancy with abnormalities that threaten their life, or cause disfigurement, the defects may challenge even expert paediatric surgeons. Many more of these babies now survive, some with heart defects (approximately 1% of all live births).

Down's Syndrome is one genetic defect often associated with congenital heart abnormalities. During pregnancy, we can now screen babies in the womb for Down's Syndrome. Genetic analyses of cells from the amniotic fluid (surrounds the baby in the womb) are used to detect the abnormality (one defect includes an extra chromosome - trisomy 21). Some foetal cardiac abnormalities are detectable during pregnancy using ultrasound. The question of survivability will become an important question. A sample of the amniotic fluid may then be required to answer it.

Down's syndrome children are special. My mother was the thirteenth child in her family. The twelfth was Polly, her Down's Syndrome older sister. My mother devoted herself to her, missing much of her schooling to care for her. Polly died when she was 18-years old, but my mother never forgot the devotion, love and affection that Polly gave to her. Even in her late nineties, any mention of Polly would still bring tears to her eyes.

Some babies with congenital heart defects cannot thrive. They may be listless and become undernourished and underdeveloped through not feeding well. They may exhibit breathlessness and their skin and lips can appear blue (cyanosed).

Blue Babies

Cyanosis is the name given to the blue coloration of the skin and lips, seen in babies who have too much de-oxygenated (venous) blood in their circulation. This occurs because:

The main pumping chamber (the left ventricle) is underdeveloped.

Not enough blood reaches their lungs (narrowing of the right-sided pulmonary and tricuspid valves).

Because arterial blood (oxygenated) gets mixed with deoxygenated (venous) blood. This occurs when the main outlet arteries cross over one another (transposition of the great vessels) or form one tube (truncus arteriosus).

Several of the above factors can combine in any one patient.

In **Fallot's tetralogy**, four congenital abnormalities occur at once. Blood does not easily reach the lungs from the right side of the heart. The right heart pumping chamber is both thickened (hypertrophied), and obstructed. There is a hole connecting the ventricles of the heart. This diverts incoming blood from the veins into the main circulation, causing the baby to be blue (cyanosed). In addition, the two main outlet arteries (the aorta and pulmonary artery) can override one another, allowing blood to mix further and deepen the cyanosis. Fallot's tetralogy is not uncommon in Down's Syndrome babies.

Babies without Cyanosis

In abnormalities without cyanosis, blood from veins does not get into the main (systemic) circulation. Holes in the top chamber (atrial septal defect) and those in the bottom heart chamber (ventricular septal defect), will usually let blood through the hole from left to right (the left side has light coloured oxygenated blood; the right side has deoxygenated, darker venous blood). It is of little consequence that left-sided oxygenated blood gets into the right side of the heart, but when right-sided blood gets across into the left side, cyanosis appears. This happens when right-sided pressures increase for some reason (as in pulmonary hypertension, when high blood flow and pressure affect the lung circulation).

A defect in the aorta that connects the arch of the aorta to one pulmonary artery leading to the lungs is called a **patent ductus**. This small connecting artery is present in every baby at birth. In all but a few cases it closes soon after birth. When it fails to close, blood flows through it, raising the pressure in the pulmonary circulation. The result is a loud murmur that occurs as the heart contracts, continuing even as it relaxes. The patent ductus needs to be closed if irreversible high pulmonary artery pressure (pulmonary hypertension) is to be avoided.

Diagnosis

We can confirm these congenital heart defects using ultrasound, MRI scanning, and heart catheterisation. The anatomy of the defects needs to be understood and their severity estimated before advising any intervention.

Some defects in babies remain undiagnosed, only to be discovered by doctors when the patient is older. These defects are then referred to as **adult congenital heart disease**.

Inheritance and the Heart

Family History

Every road and building needs a development plan before con-struction starts, and each of us inherits a set of genetic plans that serve a similar purpose. Like most plans, they will be subject to deletions, additions and transformations (mutations) as time goes by. Taking a family history is one simple way to access our inherited genetic pre-dispositions, although the accuracy of the information and its com-pleteness are sources of error.

The family history of patients with coronary heart disease and high blood pressure is often striking. Without a family history, the oppo-site applies; when there is no history of these conditions in a family, few will develop high blood pressure, heart attacks or angina, even if their symptoms suggest them. How reliable is the family history in predicting coronary artery disease and hypertension in any patient? In my experience, it helps in 75% of cases (tossing a coin is helpful in only 50% of cases, so it beats guessing or being guided by something not connected).

If a patient has one parent with coronary heart disease or high blood pressure, one in four of their children are likely to develop the same disease as their life progresses. If both parents have the condition, at least eight out of ten of their children can expect to inherit it. These are the impressions I am left with after taking thousands of family histories over a fifty-year period.

My experience suggests that the 'furring' of arteries (atherosclerosis, the cause of coronary artery disease), and the arterial muscle growth associated with hypertension, are both strongly inherited. It is now popular to think that heart disease is caused by 'unhealthy' lifestyles and diet. I beg to differ. Although they may not cause these diseases, changes in lifestyle and diet can benefit their progress. For those who have had a heart attack, eating a Mediterranean diet can reduce the chance of a second one by 70% (compared to control subjects who do not change their diet). Similar benefits apply to exercise and smoking cessation. These positive notions bring comfort to those who feel the need for control in their lives.

Without inheriting any of the adverse genes that lead to heart disease, few will develop them, whatever they eat or do.

So ask yourself this,

'Have I inherited heart disease?'

If you think you have, because it runs in your family, take heart screening seriously (read the next chapter). To find out what to do, and how to do it, go to Chapter 12. There I describe how to help yourself.

How Does Inheritance Work?

Strings of genetic instructions (genes) make up the chromosomes that sit in the nucleus of every cell we have - all 30 trillion of them. Humans have 23 pairs of chromosomes formed from just four specific amino acids (protein building blocks). Genes act as strings of instructions which direct all the various biochemical actions within our cells. They are made from a series of only four amino acids, labelled A-T-C-G, to represent A=adenine. T=thymine, C=cytosine and G=guanine. A gene code might look something like this: ACC-GATTAGGCGAGATATGC. Genetic research aims to identify the important codes, and to work out how they translate into actions within the cells. Many codes that lead to disease have already been identified, but there is a long road ahead.

Much of the code on chromosomes is redundant; a bit like a large book with gobbledegook filling most of its pages. Mutations occur when the strings of code are added to, or are deleted. Some will critically change the instructions given to cells; this can cause malfunctioning or disease. Because viruses are made from genetic material (RNA or DNA), and find their way into our cells, they have the potential to effect the critical genetic instructions responsible for making our cells work healthily. Fortunately, most viruses have only transient effects.

Two strands of chromosomes made from DNA, make up each of our 46 chromosomes (two strings of 23). At the atomic level, the two strings spiral in parallel, forming a double helix (like a bedspring made from two parallel spirals rather than one).

When cells divide, only one string from each chromosome will end up in each cell. Within each new cell, the string is used to generate another matching string. The new string is not a copy because each 'A' has to be matched by a new 'T', and each 'C' by a new 'G' (a process called replication). James Watson (born in California), and Francis

Crick (born in Northamptonshire, UK), working in Cambridge in the 1940s and 1950s, worked out how the strings of genes replicate after cell division. They published their Nobel prizewinning work in 1953.

At conception, it is a matter of chance which of the two strings of DNA from each parent the baby will get. Although there are two strings of DNA in each male sperm cell, and two in each female egg (4 strings in all), babies only get two strings; one from the father and one from the mother. If one of these strings is encoded for heart disease, there will have been a 4:1 chance of the resulting offspring getting that disease. By chance alone, one in four of the children will inherit the same heart disease as one parent. The chance of two separate offspring inheriting the same heart disease from one parent is 16:1 (4 x 4). It really is, all a matter of chance. If both parents have heart disease (high BP or artery 'furring'), not all the children will inherit it, but chances are that the majority will.

We inherit some diseases through the RNA found in cell mito-chondria (microscopic structures within every cell). These structures are responsible for energy production in the cell, and have their own genetic code. These little biochemical power plants are inherited only from the mother's ovum. That is because the father's sperm contains no mitochondria, and therefore, no mitochondrial RNA (sperm has only paternal DNA). The mitochondrial diseases are inherited only from the mother, and can cause defects in energy metabolism. We know them to be associated with heart rhythm problems and heart muscle disease.

Each genetic 'instruction' (gene) performs in a certain way. Some have a strong influence (dominant), others a weak influence (reces-sive). When animals mate, the offspring receives a mixture of their parents' genes, dictated purely by chance. The dominant ones will usually be expressed, while the weak recessive ones may remain unrevealed. This will be the case unless the child receives two recessive genes (and no dominant ones), one from each parent. The recessive gene characteristic will then become apparent. Many heart disease genes are dominant, and we need only one dominant gene to pass the disease on to our children (to one in four of our offspring on average).

Austrian monk Gregor Mendel was first to point out how all this worked (he published his work in 1866). He grew over 30,000 pea plants and observed the colour of their flowers and other features that resulted from different pollinations. He noted the plants that came from the cross-pollination of different pairs (different hybrids). He studied plant features other than colour, noting seed size and stem length. He discovered each feature to be independent of all the others.

Mendel discovered that purple coloured pea flowers dominated, and would override the white flower characteristic (a recessive trait). At the time he knew nothing about genes, but we can now look back and understand what was actually going on. We now know that only plants with two recessive (white) genes become white. Whenever the dominant purple gene is present, the resulting flowers will always be purple. This is Mendel's law of dominance brought into the modern age.

Charles Darwin published his work on evolution three years after Mendel's work. In 1900, Mendel's work was rediscovered, but had been ignored until then. Darwin never learned about the genius of Mendel's work, and the scientific insight it provided. Had he known, he might have better understood the process of evolution.

Heart Genes

Beware of companies selling genetic profile testing.

Genetic testing can be appropriate for those with a family history of heart disease, some with heart symptoms, and those with a verified heart abnormality.

The relevance of genetic testing for patients is work in progress. We have identified relevant genes in the following conditions:

Congenital Heart Disease

Down's Syndrome

Fragile X syndrome

Turner syndrome

Jacobsen syndrome

Williams syndrome

Valve and Structural Defects

Some holes in the heart (ASD and VSD)

Some cases of pulmonary valve stenosis, and

Heart muscle disease (HOCM)

Marfan syndrome

Ehlors Danlos syndrome

Heart Muscle Disease

There are at least 15 variants of the cardiomyopathy HOCM (heart muscle disease) to look for. Many have a dominant gene status.

Electrical Instability and Tachycardia Problems

Brugada syndrome

Long QT syndrome

Arrhythmic right ventricle

Ventricular Tachycardia

If a doctor has given you any of these diagnoses, ask them if your genetic profiling and that of your family is appropriate.

Heart Screening

Those with a family history of heart disease should consider the following actions:

Regular screening to detect high blood pressure and raised blood cholesterol (looking for those with a high LDL, and low HDL).

Occasional ultrasound screening, looking for artery 'furring' (every two to five years).

Echocardiography for those over 50-years old. Especially for those who have noticed shortness of breath.

In these ways, we can detect the commonest forms of heart disease and manage them for our future benefit.

Once any form of heart problem is discovered, doctors have many forms of intervention available to help, if appropriate. It is the job of medical science to determine whether any suggested intervention is likely to affect patients. What we want to do is reduce future medical events (reducing morbidity), and lengthen life expectancy (reducing mortality). If they do not help the majority, we will think them pointless, and not recommend them. New interventions have to await the accumulation of enough evidence to judge them useful and safe. Adopting them early can be a gamble worth taking if they appear harmless (like taking vitamins, nutrients, and making lifestyle changes).

When you judge a new trend, or advice about what will be good for you, use a simple scientific principle. Never allowed yourself to be fooled. Don't rely entirely on user reviews. The promises made about something new and wonderful often lack any independent confirmatory evidence. It could be a waste of time to follow them.

Once you have an early heart problem discovered, elect to have regular screening. The aim is to measure the value of any treatment or intervention you have agreed to. We do this by measuring any progression or improvement.

Regardless of making measurements and undertaking regular screening, many are likely to benefit if only they:

- Stop smoking,

- Get fit,

- Eat less dietary sodium salt,

- Boost their diet with those foods and supplements most likely to reduce the 'furring' process, and reduce blood pressure.

Who cares? We all have to die of something!

The human need for survival is strong, but so is our ability to bury our heads in the sand, hoping that our problems will go away. The fear of finding a heart problem is off-putting, and anxiety making. These are common reasons for the little interest there is in heart screening.

If there was a choice between dying and having a painless heart test, who would refuse the painless test?

I have heard people say, 'You have to die of something!' or 'I'll take what comes!' Hope, optimism, and getting on with life can promote survival. Some patients, however, have no wish to live much longer. Their aim is to survive the day, not to live to an old age. Among them are those whose life is a continuous struggle; those who are lonely, depressed and suffering despite all we can do for them.

Unless a family member or best friend has died recently with heart trouble, few will give much thought to discovering their own risks. Because those with high blood pressure or 'furred' arteries may have no symptoms, only the minority will be prompted to take action and get tested.

Is there any reason NOT to look before you leap? What would you sooner do? Look for trouble and prevent it, or let trouble continue to develop unhindered? We are not all wise enough to check the petrol in our car, our tyre pressures, or our water and oil levels before setting off on a long road trip. I have heard some say, 'Your problem is, you worry too much!'

My friend and colleague, Dr. David Baxter, developed a theory to explain human survival strategy, based on genetic profile. Our forefathers were hunter-gatherers, used to taking life as it came. Planning was not their thing. They simply did the same thing every day of their lives, while others put down roots and became villagers. The emergence of wheat (perhaps by mutation) from what was once inedible grass, made this possible. Some humans evolved a plan. That was to create a farm, build a dwelling, and develop security for their future. These people were unlike the hunter-gatherers. They gave thought to their future risks, and how they might reduce them. David Baxter observed that the same types exist today. My experience in medical practice confirms his ideas.

How do you lead your life?

Nomad style, doing the same thing every day, and always hoping for the best?

Or, do you plan your life while investing in your future?

After 10,000 years of lifestyle changes, social status has become one of the strongest predictors of disease risk. Those with the highest social status (those who plan their future and achieve what they regard as success), have only 20% of all heart attacks. Those who take life as it comes, suffer 80% of them. Is it because they are less likely to think about future risks and how to avoid them? Is it more diet related and influenced by smoking and exercise? Is it stress related or caused by a feeling of too little control over personal circumstances and security? Research studies have shown all these to be important.

We are born with some ability to assess risk, but it takes time to develop. To hope for the best, and plan for the worst may be wise, but not all of us put this into practice. After any catastrophe, analysis often reveals that arrogance and ignorance were at work. Smokers, alcoholics and drug addicts are more likely to ignore the risks. Addicts in particular may have a genetic predisposition to avoid necessary action. Some have fewer connections between their right and left brain. They have poor connections between those parts of the brain that deal with logic and information processing, and those areas which process emotional matters. They will recognise when they are taking risks, but are less inclined than most to help themselves.

What to expect when being screened.

A thorough medical history is essential, so you need to be asked if you have experienced:

- Chest pain.

- Palpitation.

- Shortness of breath.

- Ankle swelling.

- Tiredness, fatigue, and

- Blackouts

Your past, family and drug history must follow.

Taking a history can be challenging, especially when a doctor is faced with someone reluctant to be examined, or scared of what he might find. Some withhold information for personal reasons.

Next your doctor will examine you. This should include your body weight and body mass index (BMI). We will need to feel your pulse, listen to your heart and lungs, and examine your neck for vein and artery pulses (carotid arteries supply blood to the brain). Your blood pressure should be taken with a cuff appropriate to the size of your arm. We will usually take it at the beginning and end of the examination. For all those over 40-years old, an abdominal examination is important (to detect an aneurysm), and for our leg pulses to be felt.

Investigations. Next come those tests needed to follow-up any diagnostic clues found so far. Testing can unexpectedly uncover hidden forms of heart disease that could produce symptoms later on.

We often ask for **blood tests** routinely, although few will detect the presence of heart disease. There are exceptions. For patients with chest pain, we have tests that are capable of detecting heart cell damage after a heart attack.

There are several tests that determine the population risk of coronary heart disease (from averages in large groups). These include blood fats, homocysteine, clotting and inflammatory markers. Their diagnostic value in individuals, however, is far less certain.

The most important blood tests, in relation to heart screening are:

Blood lipids: Cholesterol with its subcomponents LDL and HDL, lipoprotein 'a', and homocysteine. A free fat (triglyceride) measure is usually included. It is raised in diabetics, and in those who are overweight and unfit (this combination is referred to as the 'Metabolic Syndrome'. Its presence adds to the statistical risk of coronary artery disease occurrence).

Enzymes make chemical reactions work faster within cells. They are released into the blood with heart cell damage (heart attack, etc).

Clotting risk factors (fibrinogen, Leiden factor V, etc.)

Tests for **diabetes** include blood sugar, and HbA1c (an averaging test for the amount of glucose sugar attached to red cells). Not all diabetics have artery 'furring', and only a few with 'furred' arteries have diabetes. Insulin production together with glucose and fat metabolism, provide a link to artery 'furring'.

With age, our insulin molecules change their 3-D structure; they become less effective when lowering blood sugar and fat. Before diabetes becomes obvious, some otherwise fit people will have a raised blood sugar (glucose). Defective insulin molecules can be the cause. We refer to this as **pre-diabetes**. We can discover it by performing a glucose tolerance test (repeated blood glucose tests after a 50-gram glucose drink).

Tests for inflammation. Some believe that tests of inflammation are of value (ESR, CRP) since 'furring', or atherosclerosis, is an inflammatory process. This may hold true for large groups, but is of little use as a diagnostic tool for individuals. I prefer to look for artery 'furring' directly, and not to second guess it by relying on indirect tests like blood cholesterol. For over twenty years I used carotid artery ultrasound for this purpose. This is a superior test for individual evaluation. The direct detection of artery 'furring' is far too important to ignore.

An ECG. We usually include this electrical test routinely. It reveals the electrical activity of the heart. What appears on an ECG is only indirectly related to problems with heart muscle strength and coronary blood flow (when the coronary arteries are narrowed). Because it is an electrical test, it cannot always reflect physical heart problems (heart failure, and heart contraction problems). For those with palpitations and heart rhythm problems (and for those with faintness and blackouts), a **24-48 hour ECG** can be helpful. Heart rhythms that occur only occasionally may be revealed. Those with rarer, specific electrical abnormalities, will need to have internal ECG recordings (**electrophysiology**).

An Exercise Test is essential for assessing the mechanical efficiency of the heart pump. We can observe a lot while a patient is exercising. Unfitness and unusual shortness of breath soon become apparent. Sometimes chest pain and faintness occur; they will put an early end to the test. An ECG, recorded at the same time as exercise, is an essential part of the test (to detect waveform changes and rhythm disturbances). Because of physical disability, some patients cannot perform the test.

A Chest X-ray (CXR) is now optional. We were once afraid to miss lung problems. A chest X-ray can be quite informative in certain types of heart trouble. It is essential for those with shortness of breath and heart failure.

There are many **optional tests**. If a patient has angina, has had a heart attack in the past or has a family history of coronary artery disease, I would scan their carotid arteries looking for the 'furring' process (the cause of angina and heart attacks). Its presence in the neck arteries makes 'furring' in other arteries more likely. It was obvious from my research that 'furring' did not reliably correlate to the patient's blood cholesterol or LDL cholesterol level. It correlated better to their HDL cholesterol. High levels of HDL are not often found in those with artery 'furring'. (see the Appendix for an explanation).

Once we find 'furred' arteries, those patients with a family history, but no signs of past or present disease, should be further tested. I would always advise a CT scan of the heart, looking for calcium inclusions in the coronary artery walls (a **coronary calcium score**). Those with angina should have a **CT angiogram or coronary angiogram** to assess the severity of their coronary artery 'furring', and their need for artery stenting or coronary bypass surgery (CABG).

Echocardiography is an essential test for all those with high blood pressure (to detect heart muscle hypertrophy or muscle thickening). It is essential for all those with heart murmurs, palpitations, and anyone with a family history of heart trouble.

One aim of heart screening is to discover problems before the patient notices them. Over five decades, this worked well for my patients. It often surprised me when I found heart and artery problems in otherwise healthy people. I used it to assess heart problems and to track any progress.

Over the course of 50 years, I found many 'normal', asymptomatic people, with severe coronary heart and valvular heart disease. It has not been possible in one professional lifetime, however, to prove the advantages of cardiac screening. Many of my 'pre-patients' subsequently needed an intervention such as coronary artery stenting, coronary bypass surgery or pacing. My experience of patients, decades before any of these interventions were available (in the 1960s and '70s), left me in little doubt that my cardiac screening program advantaged patients. Without early detection, a few cases of severe 'furring' would have died without warning. Some of those we did not get to screen were diagnosed later once their condition had progressed enough to produce symptoms.

Screening is expensive, and at present far too expensive for the NHS to provide (for every 40-year-old and older). The cost of saving a life, or improving the average quality of life through screening, is not always considered affordable by government agencies (breast and prostate screening are exceptions). My patients sought my advice because they disagreed with this generalised impersonal approach. My patients, however, were rich enough and forward looking enough, to want to exercise their own life-saving strategies.

In my practice I experienced an enormous advantage: long-term, patient continuity. I saw many of my patients annually or biannually, for over 40 years. This allowed me enough personal knowledge of them to spot early clinical changes, to make early diagnoses, and to plan their individual management based on their personal circumstances.

My research findings and experience, always supported the management advice I gave. The mutual trust I developed with my patients, sanctioned me to use the art of medicine alongside medical science. What my patients continued to want from me was advice tempered by my experience and my personal knowledge of them and their circumstances. Most cardiologists achieve much with one-off, impersonal consultations, but patient satisfaction and trust can be wanting. Only by establishing trusting relationships, and knowing patients well enough, can we formulate the best individual advice for patients. This is an important aspect of the art of medicine. With a patient's life at stake, applying this art will be crucial to achieving a satisfactory experience for each patient. In my book, 'The Doctor's Apprentice. The Art and Science of Medicine', I examine patient doctor relationships in detail.

Patients should insist that their doctors apply the latest and best medical science to their case. That's the easy bit! Many patients now struggle to find a doctor willing to use clinical judgment informed by personal knowledge, namely to use the art of medicine.

HOW TO HeLP YourseLF? Are you Heart smart?

First ask yourself some key questions:

- Do I have any relevant symptoms?

- Is heart disease in my family?

- When did I last have my heart checked?

- Am I overweight?

- Am I diabetic?

- Am I unfit?

- What is my usual blood pressure?

- How can I protect my heart and arteries?

Symptoms That Count

Do I have Angina? Angina is a symptom, not a disease. It was not described recently. The English physician, William Heberden, first described it in the 18th century.

One description of angina is chest tightness or discomfort that comes with exercise. It is reproducible and predictable. Patients often know that they can induce it every time with the same exercise, like walking up the hill they know, or walking fast to their nearest post-box. It usually fades while resting after exercise.

Fearing the consequences, some patients will remain in denial. Some will avoid it by walking slower. Instead of walking around their golf course, they will use a buggy. They can then legitimately say, 'I don't get angina. It is understandable when they fear the diagnosis of angina and the medical interventions that might follow. Although understandable, it lacks common sense to leave it unchecked. Once patients know about the actual risks they face, and what can be done for them, they are less likely to leave it untreated.

Emotional situations can induce angina. Calming the situation and diffusing emotions, is easier said than done. Calming words and a sedative shot of brandy are traditional, and can help in the absence of proven heart medication, but we can do better. With stresses in their background, patients will get angina much sooner on exercise. It will also come sooner in cold weather, and after eating.

I was sitting in my car with my friend Kenny. His telephone rang. It was his daughter bearing bad news. She had booked to get married in Goa, but could not afford to pay for him to attend. It was then he first experienced an attack of angina.

John Hunter was a famous 18th century surgeon, working at St. George's Hospital, London. He once said, "My life is in the hands of anyone who cares to annoy me". Being irascible and easily annoyed, he died during a hospital board meeting.

Angina is felt not only across the chest, but occasionally in the neck and upper arm. Breathlessness, fatigue, and a feeling of impending doom, sometimes accompany it. When it occurs at rest (severe) it can be mistaken for indigestion or heartburn.

Coronary artery disease is the usual cause of angina (the coronary arteries are 'furred', blocking the normal blood flow). There are exceptions, but they are rare.

Getting angina confirmed as a symptom is a matter of some urgency. Ignoring it can expose the patient to a heart attack risk; a risk that medical intervention can avert.

We have tests to confirm angina and its cause. An ECG and an exercise ECG test are both essential. Carotid (neck artery) ultrasound is useful to detect any individual 'furring' tendency (always a widespread process within the body). Most patients with coronary artery disease have 'furring' in their neck arteries (over 95% of them in my personal, 20-year experience). CT scanning and coronary arteriography will detect the 'furring', and any limitation to flow within the coronary arteries. A coronary angiogram will define the problem more accurately. All this information will help decide whether coronary vein by-pass grafting or stenting should be considered.

Am I having a heart attack?

If you feel ill, or faint, and have had chest tightness, you must ask whether or not you have had or are having a heart attack. Telephone the emergency services, because the sooner you get treated, the better are your chances of a safe outcome.

By 'heart attack' we mean the death of some heart tissue (cardiac infarction). Those who have had a heart attack always have 'furred' arteries with clot formation that blocked the flow of blood to their heart tissue.

Ninety-five percent of all heart attacks go undetected. It is important to know that chest pain is not the only symptom. Other symptoms are: feeling suddenly unwell, noticing breathlessness and feeling faint. An ECG, or heart tracing, will not always detect small heart attacks.

Shortly after diagnosing a heart attack we can give 'clot busting' treatment. Thereafter, the anticoagulants we usually give can stop further clotting. We can also perform emergency artery stenting procedures that will unblock an artery narrowing and improve blood flow. Cholesterol-lowering, 'anti-furring' 'statin' treatment, will then be advised. The 'statin' drugs most commonly used are simvastatin, atorvastatin and rosuvastatin. They vary in price and effectiveness. They can all have side-effects that vary considerably between patients. Muscle pains and bowel symptoms are the commonest. They can, however, stop the progress of artery 'furring'.

After a heart attack it is essential to measure the progress of the artery 'furring' present. This will later serve as a measure of 'statin' treatment efficacy. The aim is to keep the 'furring' process at bay. This is yet to be done routinely by doctors. Their focus is still on lowering blood cholesterol, although this is many times removed from the real problem: artery 'furring' (atherosclerosis). An annual exercise test, carotid ultrasound, and blood tests are appropriate for all those who have had a heart attack. If there is any suggestion of a murmur or heart failure, an echocardiogram will become necessary.

I am experiencing arm pain. Could it mean I have heart disease?

A slipped disc in the neck can cause arm pain. Pain from a prolapsed (slipped) disc can occur spontaneously due to age degeneration or be triggered by accidents involving the neck. Although they mostly occur as part of the aging process, engaging in sports like running and weight lifting can affect them.

While it is rare to get arm pain as an isolated heart attack symptom, some patients experience angina in their chest and in their upper arms and shoulders at the same time. This will usually accompany physical exertion or highly emotional moments. If you have a family history of heart disease and get chest tightness and arm pain together, get tested for coronary artery disease.

I have a murmur. What might be the significance?

Heart murmurs arise from narrowed or leaky valves. In addition, holes in the heart can make prolonged whooshing sounds. We can evaluate these with echocardiography (ultrasound of the heart itself). Murmurs vary in significance from 'physiological' (minor, and of no medical consequence) to serious (causing heart failure or the risk of it).

I have been stressed lately. Can it lead to heart disease?

Stress is not the cause of any disease, but causes many unhealthy bodily changes which can lead to medical problems. It can induce the onset of high blood pressure, inappropriate hormone release, clotting, reduced immunity and prolonged tiredness. These can then lead to tissue damage or disease. Reduced immunity, for instance, can lead to pneumonia. It is important to note that these responses to stress are likely to have a genetic basis, and not all of us will be prone to them. There is no standard response to stress; some of us are resistant, others are not. There is no such thing as biological equality.

In those who have coronary artery disease (many will be unaware of it unless they have been screened), stress might trigger clot formation in a coronary artery. If a heart artery gets blocked, and life-giving blood cannot reach the heart tissues through alternative routes, a heart attack can occur.

Many patients who become fatigued have battled with long-term stress. Their angina can become more intense as a result (come sooner or more frequent), and less easily managed. The same applies to those with hypertension. Stress can make high blood pressure more resistant to treatment.

While stress itself does not cause disease, it can certainly exacerbate any existing conditions. This applies not only to cardiovascular problems but also to migraine and eczema.

Stress can contribute to the commonest symptom of all: tiredness. Chronic tiredness, from a lack of restorative sleep, was observed by Florence Nightingale. She noticed that soldiers injured soon after arriving in the Crimea, had wounds that healed quickly. Those exposed to the harsh conditions for a long time, experienced wound infections that spread, often with fatal consequences.

It is essential to recognise the potential consequences of stress to some people. Stress can seriously affect their well-being and easing it can become a matter of urgency.

Have I had a Blackout?

If you have had a blackout – an event where you completely lost consciousness - you may not be fully aware of what happened. We may have to rely on the reports of others to learn what happened. Heart rhythm changes, fainting, and epilepsy, all cause blackouts. Those with fainting and epilepsy are usually aware of their problem; those with sudden onset rhythm changes may be mystified by what caused them to black out without warning.

For those who have experience less than complete unconsciousness, the diagnosis may not be as straightforward as it seems. Both vertigo (head spinning sensation) and fainting can unsettle and disorientate patients, and be more perplexing than actual blackouts. Vertigo arises from a disturbance of the delicate balance mechanisms in the inner ear.

Fainting is a reflex response that leads gradually to diminished consciousness in response to a painful or shocking event. Low blood pressure is a predisposing factor, especially in hot weather when more salt is lost in sweat. Salt will elevate high blood pressure further, but can help elevate the blood pressure of fainters. Those who lose salt easily, and have low blood pressure, may be prone to fainting if they restrict their dietary salt intake. The prerequisite for taking extra sodium salt is having a consistently low BP (110mms Hg or less) with no known tendency to high blood pressure.

Those subject to fainting or epilepsy usually get a warning (but not always). Faintness can begin with nausea, pallor (pale skin) and sweating. Observers will see them become pale and sweaty. At the same time they will usually have a slow pulse and low blood pressure. Most adult epileptics are aware of their pre-existing condition.

A very slow pulse (life-threatening heart block that needs a pacemaker), and life-threatening, rapid electrical heartbeat activity (ventricular tachycardia or fibrillation), will cause sudden blackouts. We can save the lives of these patients by implanting a defibrillation device. Patients most at risk from these life-threatening heart rhythms are those with heart failure and heart muscle disease.

At my age surely I can expect to feel a little breathless?

That may be true for many with medical problems (lung disease and anaemia), but the cause always needs to be questioned.

Why am I breathless?

- Being overweight and unfit, are the commonest causes. Let's consider them.

- If you are overweight, losing a minimum of seven pounds (3.2 Kgs), should noticeably improve your breathlessness.

How can I improve my fitness?
- Walk to improve your fitness.

- Slowly increase your walking distance.

- Stop when fatigued.

- Gradually increase your walking speed, but stop when fatigued (whatever your fitness level).

Later on, use this interval technique: walk fast until you get breathless, then rest or walk slowly until you get your breath back. Repeat this fast/slow process and you will slowly notice improvement. Over 10 days, you should be able to walk further and faster than you did before getting breathless.

Exercise can delay the appearance of coronary disease. If you have coronary disease, it may slow its progress. It can even help those with heart failure, although it would be wrong for them to push their exercise too hard. We must all keep our exercise within the limits of our fatigue. There is no benefit in exercising beyond the point of fatigue. Pushing yourself beyond these limits is for athletes in training only.

How often should I exercise?

To begin with, a minimum of three times each week, increasing only when you feel up to it. To begin with, you will get muscle pains. These will take a day or two to subside. Don't aggravate your muscles, it will hold back your progress. Better to exercise again once your muscles have recovered.

Those who prefer **weight training** should limit their repetitions to those which bring them weakness and/or breathlessness. Do not go beyond these limits; you could injure your muscles and put your progress back.

My breathlessness is getting worse. Should I worry?

Breathlessness is a common early feature of coronary artery disease, even for those who are fit. If you notice it in association with chest tightness, be concerned. If your weight has not increased, your health has not changed, and you do not have asthma or a chest infection, get yourself checked for coronary artery disease (especially if you are over 40-years of age and have a family history of heart disease).

I have Chest Pain. Should I worry?

Is your pain angina?Pain is often the wrong word. Those who have angina describe it as tightness, not pain.Remember that angina is usually be brought on by exercise, and by the same amount of exercise each time. It is often associated with breathlessness. The discomfort is not continuous; it usually disappears gradually once exercise stops.

Try twisting your torso around in several directions. Does this make your chest hurt? Try taking deep breaths. Does that make your chest hurt? If so, the pain is more likely to come from your chest wall. Muscle and cartilage pain are more common than angina, especially in those who do little exercise. Chest wall pain tends to be sharp or continuous, rather than just on exercise. Chest wall or musculoskeletal chest pain will not usually get worse with exercise unless an injured muscle is involved.

Try pressing over the painful areas. If any are tender, some of your tissues may be inflamed. Anti-inflammatory drugs (many cause indigestion) and exercise (like press-ups), could help.

I have calf muscle pain every time I walk the same distance. What should I do?

It sounds as if you have **claudication**, a pain (or tightness) in the calf muscles caused by diminished blood flow to the muscles. Like angina, 'furring' and narrowing within the leg arteries is the cause (sometimes caused by 'furring' in the arteries of the abdomen or pelvis).

A few patients get angina and claudication together, with widespread 'furring' in many arteries. We refer to such patients as an **arteriopath** (those who have pathological 'furring' in many arteries). Symptoms will appear first from the most blocked artery. Some patients with leg artery narrowing may not walk far enough, or fast enough, to get angina.

Ultrasound testing of the arteries and veins in the legs and lower abdomen needs to be done.

Sometimes, leg pain results from vein clotting (**deep vein thrombosis**), or vein inflammation (**thrombophlebitis**), rather than an artery problem. Vein inflammation can bind any clots to the vein wall, making them less likely to break loose and travel to the lungs (pulmonary embolism). A blood test for clotting (D-Dimer), with an ultrasound scan of the leg veins, provide a useful diagnostic combination.

My heart sometimes beats fast. Could it be serious?

Palpitation is the name we give to an awareness of the heart beating. The seriousness of palpitation depends on the heart rhythm causing it.

Many people feel their heart racing or skipping beats. It will sometimes beat irregularly. Some fear that their heart will stop. This disconcerting feeling can induce anxiety and panic. Fortunately, such reactions are mostly inappropriate since palpitations are most often caused by innocent extra beats. Unfortunately, anxiety can make palpitations worse.

Apart from innocent extra beats, the commonest causes of palpitation are abnormal heart rhythm disturbances. They are:

Supraventricular (atrial) tachycardia (fast beating).

Ventricular tachycardia, and

Atrial fibrillation (more often in those over 50-years old).

Atrial fibrillation is a common, potentially serious problem, usually found in people over 50-years old (Read more about it in Chapters 1 & 6)

Without capturing an ECG or 24-hour ECG recording, it leaves us to guess the origin of any palpitation. Sometimes they can only be recorded while the patient is asleep. Sometimes they occur during exercise. They are then thought to be serious.

A few will need further evaluation with electrophysiological testing (recordings from inside the heart). There is some good news for those who need it. Those with re-entry tachycardia (inherited extra electrical pathways) can be treated at the same time (catheter ablation). This is a safe and efficient way to eliminate the problem (using radio-frequency electromagnetic waves, or cold catheter techniques – cryoablation).

My feet swell. Is my heart weak?

Swollen feet occur in those who sit a lot. Swollen feet can cause alarm, and are sometimes a sign of heart failure. Fortunately, that is much less common than prolonged sitting as a cause. When the heart is weak and unable to pump adequately, the feet usually swell.

Deciding the cause can be difficult for doctors. Heart failure is easily missed, and that is serious because it can reduce the life expectancy of those left untreated (the prognosis is the same as some cancers). When the cause of swollen feet is misdiagnosed, patients who merely sit too long, risk being treated inappropriately for heart failure.

Heart Failure as a cause of swollen feet: The diagnosis of a weak heart can be confirmed by physical examination (my preference), blood testing (BNP or proBNP - blood natriuretic peptide), and cardiac ultrasound. Some general physicians prefer to rely on BNP or proBNP. This is a chemical found in the blood. It is made as the heart stretches and dilates, as in heart failure. A normal blood level of this chemical, effectively rules out heart failure for those unable to detect it otherwise.

Other causes of swollen feet: Swollen feet can occur in hot weather, especially in those prone to fluid retention (pregnancy and the menopause; those on the contraceptive pill, and those who are physically inactive). We often see swollen feet in those with long-term, leg vein problems.

One sided foot swelling: A one-sided, rapid onset leg swelling, can be caused by infection (cellulitis caused by a streptococcal bacterium spreading up the leg), leg injury, varicose vein inflammation, or a deep vein thrombosis (DVT, occurring during bed rest after surgery, or a prolonged illness). For women, it can start with oestrogen hormone medication (the contraceptive pill and HRT). When we suspect a DVT, a blood D-dimer test and leg ultrasound will help to make the diagnosis. Whatever the cause, a diagnosis needs to be made quickly and medical management started.

Rare causes: I have only seen two cases of lymphoedema, a rare inherited condition. Patients have permanently swollen legs from a young age. An effective treatment has yet to be found.

In conclusion, diagnosing the cause of swollen feet is crucial for effective medical management. By employing various diagnostic approaches, healthcare professionals can ensure that appropriate treatment is given to improve our patient's quality of life and life expectancy.

I am tired all the time. Is it my heart? Am I about to have a heart attack?

There are many hidden factors that contribute to heart disease.

Sleepless nights fuelled by stress, worry and concern, can cause ill-health. Poor sleep is the commonest cause of tiredness and the precursor of many health issues.

In several retrospective studies of heart attack patients, researchers found an unexpected correlation. In the year before, most slept less well. They suffered daytime tiredness, fatigue and even exhaustion, accompanied by irritability. These were all noticed by relatives and friends, who also noticed what seemed to be premature aging.

Tiredness is not a symptom specific to heart trouble. Many medical conditions can drain our bodily energy. If however, tiredness is associated with increasing breathlessness and chest tightness (or pain) on exercise, patients should consider a heart check urgent.

By taking charge of the stresses that cause our poor sleep, we can improve our quality of life and even avoid the deterioration of the medical conditions we may have.

Other issues:

Am I overweight? Does it Matter?

Here is a doctor's perspective on body weight.

In considering body weight, doctors use a calculation: the ratio of body weight and height^2. This is the Body Mass Index (BMI). To calculate it we multiply the body weight in kilograms, by the square of the height in centimetres (cms^2).

Tall people have an advantage. They can add a lot of weight before their BMI registers them as overweight. Short people need only small amounts of added body weight to register them as overweight. The accepted normal range of BMI is 18.5 to 24.9. You will be regarded as obese if your BMI is greater than 30. Those between 25 and 29.9 are called overweight. I always question the clinical relevance of these categories for individuals. They are unquestioningly relevant for large groups. I prefer to relate body weight to well-being and exercise ability.

From a statistical point of view (taken from group averages), most doctors accept overweight as a heart disease risk factor. This does not translate into a reliable risk factor for every individual; it only provides a crude guide.

More surprising is the fact that social status is a more significant risk factor for heart attack risk. Those who are relatively uneducated and on a low pay, face a three to five-fold higher chance of heart attacks and strokes than those who are educated and highly paid. We refer to this as the social divide in health; a prevalent issue in most nations. In comparison, the health impact of body weight on heart disease is much smaller (risk increased by 30% at the most).

As someone who spent many decades investigating and treating heart disease, obesity did not impress me as a common feature. The minority of those I treated with coronary artery disease were obese. Perhaps the majority of obese patients died before they came to be treated. I doubt it.

There is a paradox here that applies to all forecasting, whether it is predicting heart attacks or the weather. The general weather forecast may be for sunshine, but will this apply to you and where you live? Perhaps it's best to look out of the window and make your own prediction, rather than accept the nationwide forecast from experts? The answer, of course, is to consider both.

There is little doubt about it; overweight patients get breathless more quickly, and get angina sooner than their slimmer counterparts. Even if obesity does not itself cause heart disease, body weight is an issue for all of us. It hampers fitness and can reduce our exercise tolerance.

The word **diabetes** means to pass sugar in the urine. Diabetes causes both glucose and fat (triglyceride) to build up in the blood. Insufficient or defective insulin is the cause. When insulin is working normally, it allows glucose and fat to enter our cells. That will lower blood glucose and fat levels.

Diabetics are at risk of coronary artery disease. This is probably because the 'furring' of arteries contains fat (cholesterol, and oxidised LDL), and fat metabolism is disturbed in diabetes. Over many decades, I saw thousands of patients with artery 'furring', but few had diabetes. Perhaps they were mostly pre-diabetic, but I doubt it.

Are there foods that are good for the heart and arteries? Discovering Heart-Healthy Foods.

Apart from what food gurus tell us, what do we know for sure about food and how it affects our heart and arteries?

Animal experiments have shed light on which nutrients might promote, prevent or reduce the 'furring' process in arteries. Dietary saturated fat can definitely contribute to artery 'furring' (atherosclerosis is the process that blocks arteries). We also know that sodium salt can adversely affect blood pressure control and heart failure treatment (although useful for those with low blood pressure).

Despite the commonly voiced advice about the foods that are good or bad for us, we remain unsure about which foods might actually prevent or promote coronary artery disease and artery 'furring' in other parts of the body.

I have researched the animal experiment evidence and found the nutrients which at least protect the arteries of animals. Since arteries are primitive tubes which have not evolved much over millions of years, the results of animal experiments are likely to apply to human arteries. There is little or no direct human evidence available to rely on.

In my quest to find nutrients that might be good or bad for our arteries, I had to invent a measure; I called it the Cardiac Value™ of food. If you are interested in the details, my books on the subject (listed in About the Author) detail the 'goodies' and the 'baddies' in food. The nutrient content ratio of these two nutrient types I used to calculate my own Cardiac Value™ for each food.

While researching the subject, I came up with some surprising results. Based on their nutrient chemistry, offal and shellfish reign supreme when it comes to artery 'furring' protection. Surprisingly, sunflower oil has more protective nutrients than olive oil, and both chocolate and ice cream are the worst foods we can eat for our artery health; they contain nutrients that are likely to promote 'furring' (they are atherogenic). Quantity matters. Small portions are unlikely to do much good or harm. Eating large quantities every day is bound to have a greater effect.

Do genetics matter more than food? I think so. Can food be dangerous to those who have not inherited artery 'furring' genes? (no 'furring' on artery ultrasound studies). Again, I think so. Genetic analysis, however, has yet to provide enough information, while family history can serve as a guide.

Having identified minerals, vitamins, and amino-acids with some evidence of experimental benefit on 'furring', I wondered which foods might contain them. That is made possible by my calculations, but another challenge presents itself. That challenge is to find foods with these beneficial nutrients, but not too many calories or unhealthy nutrients. The conclusion I came to was that it is difficult to eat enough of the beneficial foodstuffs, without getting too many calories or adverse nutrients. There is perhaps a reason for this. Natural foods existed long before humans ate them, and were not designed for our health.

While the quest to understand the perfect diet for a healthy heart is complicated, exploring the subject has been an interesting journey. Since so many western middle-aged people die as a result of artery 'furring', it's a journey worth pursuing.

STILL WOrrieD ABOUT YOUr HeArT?

**PROTECTING AND CARING FOR YOUR HEART AND
ARTERIES**

A SUMMARY OF NEEDS

For those with no known risk: The minimum requirement for
personal reassurance is to rule out high blood pressure and artery
'furring'. Most doctors insist on blood cholesterol measurement, etc.,
but these are not specific enough to rule out a diagnosis of coronary
disease in individuals. A painless ultrasound scan of your neck arteries
will show whether you are 'furring' your arteries or not (the main cause
of coronary artery disease), and whether you are at risk of artery related
problems.

Even without an inherited family risk, we should all check our
blood pressure a few times every year. For those with a family history

of high blood pressure, it can change from normal to high within one year. It seems as if the controlling genes have their own time clock mechanism. I have seen this occur in women as their menopause starts. It is not so easy to predict in men.

A Minimal Cardiac Screen includes a structured questionnaire to assess family history and symptoms. Examination of the heart and arteries should be done together with your height and weight, and urine check.

Get a personal report sent to you. It should detail what was found, and what you might need to consider.

A Full Cardiac Screen involves a consultation and examination with a cardiologist (or a specially trained physician). Blood tests can assess your general health status. A neck artery ultrasound scan will show any 'furring' present (it occurs more often in the neck arteries than other arteries). An ECG exercise test will 'road-test' your heart. These are the minimum requirements.

If your problem is high blood pressure, blackouts, heart failure, or heart valve problems, a 24h ECG and an ultrasound of the heart itself (echocardiogram) are required. Taken together, these are the basic screening requirements for astronauts, and others where no compromises can be tolerated (perhaps yourself, and your nearest and dearest).

One major point to these tests is to provide a baseline for future reference. It is from this base that future changes become easily apparent, and diagnoses are made more easily.

EPILOGUE

Heart disease and cancer are the commonest killers of middle-aged people in the western world. Coronary heart disease is partly preventable, and once we know of its existence, we can do much to contain it. To do the best we can, we must find cardiovascular problems as early as possible, well before any symptoms arise.

APPENDIX

The Cause of Heart Attacks

'Furring' (atheroma or atherosclerosis) in arteries does not precipitate like snow, but is mostly formed by the tissue (endothelium) of their inner lining (the intima). The 'furring' is made of cholesterol, often mixed with scar tissue and calcium containing compounds. When one of each predominates it produces three separate types of 'furring'. The lipid-rich ones are the most dangerous. They can breakdown, ulcerate and attract artery blocking clot. The scarred and calcium-rich plaques do this much less often.

The cholesterol and calcium compounds (calcium apatite) in the artery 'furring' can be visualised early on in life (usually not before the age of 35-years), using an ultrasound device on the neck (carotid) or leg arteries. The calcium can be imaged using a CT scan. This can provide a calcium score for how much is present. This is a surrogate score for how much coronary artery disease is present.

Blood cholesterol testing is useful for predicting what will happen to populations. It is useless (a 60/40 chance of being correct) when used to predict the presence of artery 'furring', and actual heart attack risk in individuals.

Heart attacks occur when a clot forms on 'furring' that ruptures and ulcerates. This can happen quickly, giving the impression that a heart attack 'comes out of the blue'.

How can artery 'furring' be detected early?

- **Ultrasound imaging of the neck arteries** is simple, painless and quick. It can be repeated as often as necessary. If 'furring' is present in the neck arteries, it is likely to be present in other arteries like those of the heart (coronary arteries). If not present in the neck arteries, the heart arteries will only rarely be affected (1/1000 chance in my data set).

- **A CT scan (X-ray) of the heart** shows the actual presence of chalk (calcium apatite) in the arteries. A negative test means that you are very unlikely to have narrowing of your heart arteries. It will miss 'furring' that is made mainly of fat without calcium. These are thought to be the most likely to rupture.

- **Catheterisation of the heart is NOT a screening test.** It involves injecting a dye into the arteries of the heart through a tube inserted into your arm or groin, then advanced into the heart arteries. It has dangers, it is expensive, and involves a lot of X-rays. It is a must for those with exercise limiting angina, and those who have had a heart attack. It is not a test for early detection.

- **ECG Exercise tests** are an imperfect way to detect narrowed heart arteries. They are useful to observe what happens to blood pressure with exercise. A useful, simple, and inexpensive test, it will detect 85%+ of those with severely narrowed coronary arteries, but the arteries have to be quite narrowed (85% or more) before the test is expected to be positive. A treadmill exercise test is reproducible and allows the comparison of ECGs from time to time. This makes it more useful than bicycle based exercise tests.

Dying of a Broken Heart. Is this a myth? Most spouses die within 3 years of their partner.

We doctors have been backward in acknowledging the simple fact that the heart, brain and psyche are connected.

In the 17th century, William Harvey wondered why the pulse increased with emotion. He failed to find out, but wrote his findings in a famous book, *De Motu Cordis (1628)*. Doctors whose job is purely technical will focus on surgery, on the opening of arteries and valves. They perform invaluable feats of biomedical engineering. Physicians, however, need a different focus. Unfortunately William Harvey's focus has all but disappeared, but is now slowly re-emerging.

Patients need the connection between neurophysiology and cardiac physiology to be respected by medical professionals. That may entail accepting that some could die from a broken heart. Once again focussing on the art of medicine, alongside the science of medicine, would better pave the way to patient satisfaction. Patients should expect no less from those who care for them.

GLOSSARY

Heart Related Words

ACE inhibitors: Drugs that lower blood pressure and treat heart failure. Side effects: cough and impotence. See also **ARB**s.

Alpha-blocker: Drugs that dilate arteries. Used for angina and high blood pressure.

Aneurysm: Equivalent to a 'blow out' in a tyre, but in an artery. A thin bubble may appear which can rupture. Occurs in the aorta and in brain arteries (cerebral aneurysm).

Angiogram: an X-ray video taken while injecting an iodine based dye into the heart cavities or coronary arteries.

Angioplasty: a method for opening narrowed coronary arteries using a balloon catheter inserted into the heart arteries.

Aorta: The main artery leading from the heart to the body.

Aortic valve: the main outlet valve. It can get leaky (incompetence), and constricted (stenosis).

ARB: Angiotensin Re-uptake Blockers. Treatment for hypertension and heart failure.

Artery: Blood vessel tubes that carry oxygenated blood from the heart to the tissues.

Atheroma or atherosclerosis: Cholesterol, calcium and scar formation beneath the inner lining (intima) of the larger arteries.

Atrium (plural: atria): The priming, top chambers of the heart.

Atrial fibrillation: A chaotic, irregular heart rhythm, arising from the atria. There is an attendant risk of clot formation. This is one cause of strokes.

Beta-blocker: a drug that blocks the effects of adrenaline. Useful in some forms of high blood pressure and tachycardia.

Blood pressure: The pressure of the pulse, generated by the heart, within every artery. The maximum pressure reached is called the systolic pressure. The pressure between beats is the diastolic pressure.

Bradycardia: slow heart rate. Found in athletes and those with heart block.

Bruce Protocol: A standardised treadmill exercise test regime. An international standard for ECG exercise testing.

Cardiomegaly: An enlarged heart. Found in heart failure, high blood pressure, and heart valve problems.

Cardiomyopathy: Heart muscle disease. Often inherited.

Cardiovascular disease: Diseases of the heart and circulation.

Catheterisation: A method of examining the heart from the inside. A plastic tube is inserted into an artery, then advanced under X-ray control to the heart. Pressures are measured and dye injections are performed.

Cor Pulmonale: Heart failure due to severe lung disease.

Coronary: A common term for heart attack. Technically used to describe the heart's own arteries. Leonardo da Vinci thought they looked like a crown (corona) on top of the heart.

De-fibrillation: Any method that stops the heart fibrillating. Drug and electrical methods are used.

Delta-wave (δ-wave): An unusual ECG wave pattern found in people with a liability to a particular type of fast heart beat (tachycardia).

Diastole: The resting phase within the heart beat after the main pumping chamber has contracted. In this period the heart is 'primed' by the contracting atria.

Digoxin: Drug derived from the foxglove plant. It slows the heart and was once thought to improve the strength of heart contraction.

EBCT: (**E**lectron **B**eam **C**omputed **T**omogram): A CT X-ray of the heart. Shows calcium compounds in the coronary arteries. A normal result means a low risk of current coronary artery disease.

ECG: Electrocardiogram or recording of the heart's electrical activity.

Echocardiogram (echo-sounding) or ultrasound: A picture formed by ultrasonic reflections from the valves, heart chambers, and heart muscle, etc.

ECG Exercise test: An ECG taken during exercise on a treadmill or bicycle. Used to diagnose narrowed heart arteries, blood pressure variation and heart rhythm problems.

Electrophysiology: Study of the heart's electrical activity using an electrode catheter inside the heart.

Extra beats or Extrasystoles: There are two types: ventricular (from the main pumping chamber) and atrial (from the priming chamber). They are early or premature electrical impulses that give the feeling of a 'missed' or extra beat.

Fibrillation: Irregular electrical heart activity. Fatal if not corrected when arising from the main pumping chambers (ventricular fibrillation); an important issue when fibrillation occurs in the atria.

Heart attack: Death of heart tissue due to coronary artery clot formation.

Heart block: Delayed electrical transmission through heart tissue. Can cause blackouts (syncope).

Hypertension: High blood pressure. **Reactive or labile** - up and down all the time. Primary hypertension if constantly above 140 systolic (the top figure) and over 85 diastolic (the lower figure). Secondary hypertension is due to a disease (kidney damage, etc.)

Infarct: Death of tissue i.e. cardiac infarct = heart attack. They can be anterior - in the front of the heart; inferior - underneath, or posterior – behind the heart.

J-point: A specific point on the QRS wave of an ECG.

JVP: Jugular venous pulse. The fluid level of the heart. Raised in right heart failure.

Mitral valve: One of the 4 main heart valves. Mitral stenosis forms a flow restricted mitral valve – mostly the consequence of rheumatic fever.

Myocardium: The heart muscle.

Node: The sino-atrial and A-V nodes are part of the heart's electrical system.

Pericardium. The sac enveloping the heart. When inflamed it is called pericarditis. Pericardial effusion is when it becomes filled with fluid.

Pulmonary: Pertaining to the lungs.

Pulmonary hypertension - High artery pressure in the lungs.

Pulmonary oedema: Fluid in the lungs. Often from raised left heart pressures or valve blockage, like mitral stenosis.

q-wave: ECG wave. Possible sign of a previous heart attack or infarct.

r-wave: Part of the normal ECG waveform.

Reversion: Putting the heart rhythm back to normal using a DC shock.

s-wave: Follows the r-wave on an ECG.

'Sartan' drug. An ARB. Used for hypertension. Proven to prevent strokes and heart attacks.

Stenosis: Partial blockage of an artery or valve. A significant stenosis is one where the flow of blood is reduced.

t-wave: The recovery wave of the ECG.

Tachycardia: Fast heart beating. Comes in various forms: 'supraventricular' when it arises from the atria; 'ventricular' when it comes from the pumping chambers. 'Nodal' or 'junctional' when it comes from the middle part of the heart.

Tietze's Syndrome: Chest pain caused by inflamed chest wall cartilages.

Tricuspid: A valve on the right side of the heart.

Trinitrin: A tablet placed under the tongue. It dilates the coronary arteries. Used for the relief of angina.

u-wave: Follows the t-wave on ECG.

Ventricular: Pertaining to either the right or left heart pumping chamber.

Vasodilatation: The opening of small blood vessels (arterioles).

Wenckebach Phenomenon: A type of electrical delay seen on ECG.

WPW (Wolff-Parkinson-White Syndrome): A type of fast beating of the heart caused by an extra electrical pathway in the heart.

X or Syndrome X: Chest pain identical to angina but with no coronary artery disease.

ABOUT THE AUTHOR

D r David H. Dighton qualified from the London Hospital Medical College in 1966 with MB BS (London) degrees. In 1970, he became a British Heart Foundation Fellow in Cardiology at St. George's Hospital Hyde Park Corner, Central London, working with Dr Aubrey Leatham and Dr Alan Harris. In 1973 he became an MRCP(UK), and a Lecturer (London University) in General Medicine and Cardiology at Charing Cross Hospital, London. In 1980, he was appointed Chef de Clinique (Assistant Professor) at the Vrije University Hospital in Amsterdam. Having returned to the UK in1982, he worked in his own private cardiac practice, established in Loughton, Essex. In 2000 he started a private (non NHS) diagnostic cardiac centre specialising in early heart and artery disease detection and preventative cardiology.

Contact: www.daviddighton.com   email david@daviddighton.com

Other books by the author: *Eat to Your Heart's Content. The diet and lifestyle for a healthy heart.*(2003). HeartShield Ltd. ISBN:

0-9551072-0-2 ; *HeartSense. How to look after your heart.*(2006) . HeartShield Ltd. ISBN 0-9551072-1-0 ; *The NHS. Our Sick Sacred Cow. Causes and Cures (2023)* (Paperback & ebook). **In preparation are:** *The Doctor's Apprentice. The Art and Science of Medical Practice; Weight Wars; Cardiology for Students*

INDEX

www.ingramcontent.com/pod-product-compliance
Lightning Source LLC
Chambersburg PA
CBHW071233020426
42333CB00015B/1450